Hollow Crown of Fire

Hollow Crown of Fire

A Discovery of Meaning in the Coronavirus Pandemic and its Predecessors

For Meredith,
with my love!
Barbara

Barbara E. Hort, Ph.D.
Foreword by Jean Shinoda Bolen, M.D.

Published in the United States by White Horse Wordsmithing, LLC.

The views expressed in this book are the author's own, and do not purport to represent or co-opt the views of those whose work is cited. Additionally, although this work cites medical, psychological, scientific, and historical information, it is not to be construed in any way, nor on any topic, as counsel, instruction, or advice. Finally, this book presents the most current version of medical, psychological, scientific, and historical information that was available at the moment the book went to press in December 2022. However, some of this information will inevitably be expanded or even contradicted by later research, and I apologize for those unforeseeable inaccuracies. You can be sure that if my crystal ball were prescient enough to reveal which facts would become obsolete, I would be using it to prognosticate even more important matters.

ISBN (paperback): 9798986981208
ISBN (ebook): 9798986981215

Book design by Christy Day, Constellation Book Services
Cover image courtesy of Shutterstock

Manufactured in the United States of America

Library of Congress Cataloguing-in-Publication Data
Names: Hort, Barbara E., author.
Description: First Edition. |White Horse Wordsmithing, LLC. | Includes index.
Identifiers: ISBN 9798986981208 (paperback print) | ISBN 9798986981215 (ebook)
Subjects: Pandemics | Epidemics | Covid-19 Pandemic 2020- | Black Death | Influenza Epidemic 1918-1919 | Smallpox.
Classification: LCC 2022920768

This book is dedicated to the uncountable multitudes
whose lives, loved ones, and personal sense of meaning
have been devoured by the wildfires of pandemic disease.
This discovery of meaning in our major pandemics
will come too late for those poor souls, but perhaps it
will offer some comfort to the modern multitudes
whose lives are burning in the pandemic
of the novel coronavirus.

I want to express my profound gratitude
for the work of the late Alfred W. Crosby,
whose breadth of vision inspired me to believe
that such a book could be written at all,

and for the cherished support of Chris Coleman,
whose fierce enthusiasm inspired me to believe
that such a book could be written by *me*.

Contents

Foreword
by Jean Shinoda Bolen, M.D.

I have a deep respect for history because I believe that our past experience holds the answers to our present problems. Our past is not dead and buried. It is alive inside us, alive in its residue of suffering and alive in its capacity to heal. But we cannot benefit from the past until we learn what has happened and how it has affected us. This is a fundamental principle, both in psychological healing and in human history.

One of the great mysteries of historical research is that it has paid so little attention to pandemic disease. This is a tragic omission because pandemics have been one of the most powerful forces in human history. I think historians' blind spot about pandemics is part of their larger blind spot about all aspects of the Feminine, including human bodies and human feelings.

Historians have focused much more on the masculine topics of power and politics. Pandemics are about sick and dying bodies, and also our feelings of fear and grief when people are sick and dying. Pandemics change the course of history, but they don't "make history" in the usual way. They don't make speeches or mount armies. What pandemics do mostly is to make us sick and dead...and also very afraid.

Another reason that historians have said very little about pandemics is that people have understood very little about disease for most of human history and we tend to ignore or be silent about things we don't understand. As a result, human beings have had little insight into pandemic disease, even though it is one of the most important forces in human evolution.

I tell you all of this to explain why I have strongly encouraged my friend Dr. Barbara Hort to publish this book. Barbara says that she began *Hollow Crown of Fire* simply as a way to make some meaning for herself when the Covid pandemic erupted in March 2020. But now that she has agreed to share her journey in this book, we all have the opportunity (maybe for the first time ever) to derive some meaning from our painful history with pandemic disease.

In this book, Barbara takes us through the story of pandemics as if it were an enormous drama on the human stage. She uses her gifts as a Jungian psychologist and a theatrical storyteller to integrate what medicine, psychology, mythology, and history can tell us about pandemics and their effects on humankind. Barbara has thoroughly documented this complicated story, but her narrative style makes the story very accessible and even entertaining. She takes us on a journey through territory that could feel dangerous and overwhelming, except that her wisdom and clarity keep us safe. And Barbara doesn't lecture us. Instead, she lets each of us find our own points of meaning as we travel by her side.

The philosopher George Santayana once said that "Those who cannot remember the past are condemned to repeat it." I would add that if we don't learn from the past, we will lose what it has to teach us. That would be a terrible loss. Indeed, we have already paid a high price for the centuries of insight that we have lost about pandemic disease. Barbara is giving us a chance to redeem that loss. Because of this book, we can retrieve the wisdom of our pandemic past so that we can be better prepared for our pandemic present...and our pandemic future.

I hope that many people will read *Hollow Crown of Fire* and take advantage of the hard work that Dr. Barbara Hort has done for us. It is time for us to redeem our history of pandemic suffering. Those of us who accompany Barbara on this journey will be able to reap the benefits of learning from our pandemic experience—benefits that include a renewed sense of meaning and hope.

PROLOGUE

Why Should We Bother to Look for the Meaning of a Pandemic?

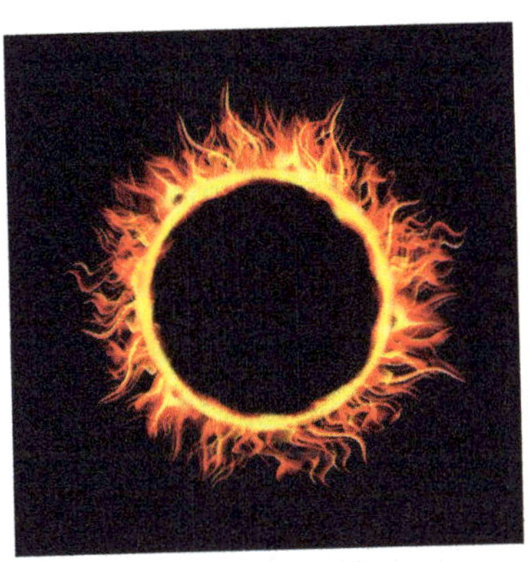

Nothing can we call our own but death...
...For within the Hollow Crown
That rounds the mortal temples of a king
Keeps Death his court and there the Antic sits,
Scoffing his state and grinning at his pomp,
Allowing him a breath, a little scene
To monarchize, be fear'd and kill with looks,
Infusing him with self and vain conceit.
As if this flesh which walls about our life
Were brass, impregnable. And humour'd thus,
Comes at the last and with a little pin
Bores through his castle wall. And farewell, king!

– **William Shakespeare,** *Richard II*, III.ii

"Nothing can we call our own but death."

Death is the inescapable consequence of life. Saints and sociopaths, movie stars and murderers—every one of us must accept a lethal pinprick from the Antic named Death. Most of us will experience a rather anonymous death, unless we are some rarely famous person, or unless our death occurs in some famous catastrophe. But famous victims only come from our famous catastrophes of war and natural disaster. Until recently, our catastrophes of pestilence have received hardly a glance from humankind. Our pandemics have been given minimal attention as compared to other historical events, events that were deemed by historians (and sometimes by the people of their own era) to deserve more attention than the deadly disease that was incinerating the populace.

The result has been that people who have died in pandemics have died unseen. Unseen and also unsung, except by a few traumatized survivors of the scourge. This is tragic because it is generally believed that more people have died of pestilence than of all wars and natural disasters combined. Consider the fact that within the year March 2020 to March 2021, more Americans died of Covid-19 than died in World War I, World War II, Vietnam, and 9/11 *combined*. And yet, the people who have died in pandemics have been shunned like the diseases that killed them—contaminated and contaminating, terrified and terrifying. They have been isolated and condemned by their fellow humans, subjected to hideous suffering and dumped into anonymous graves. They have had no understanding of the thing that was destroying their world, and most tragically, they have frequently been led to believe that they brought their anguish upon themselves.

In the end, nearly all the victims of pandemic disease have succumbed to a terrible death, or permanently lost their health, or watched their loved ones die in anguish, and all without a wisp of meaning for their misery. Admittedly, the meaning in much of our suffering eludes us. But given the extremes of agony, terror, and despair that are inflicted by pandemic disease, it is especially heartbreaking that nearly all of its victims have died without any personal sense of meaning.

And let's be clear: Just because the meaning of something is not *easy* to find, that doesn't mean it *can't* be found. The real challenge in finding the meaning of a thing, especially a confounding thing, is that meaning can only be defined and discovered by the person who seeks it. No other person can define for us the meaning of our life, our death, or anything else. Each of us must consider the story whose meaning we seek, and then decide for ourselves where its meaning lies, regardless of whether that story is as sweet as a kiss or as monstrous as a global pandemic.

At this point, you may be wondering why it's important to make meaning at all. If humanity has persevered through millennia of meaningless death from pandemic disease, why bother changing things now? After all, it has been centuries since the Buddhists declared that all life must entail suffering. But then the Swiss psychoanalyst Carl Jung observed that our suffering is only made bearable by our ability to derive meaning from it. And centuries before Jung declared that truth, William Shakespeare was bringing it to life on the stage. Shakespeare told stories that gave meaning to suffering by providing some context for its mad despair...and its poignant courage.

It is regrettable that Shakespeare is not alive to capture the essence of the current pandemic in one of his astounding plays. But then, Shakespeare probably wouldn't write about the coronavirus, even if he were living here with us. There was an active pandemic raging while Shakespeare was writing about "the Hollow Crown that rounds the mortal temples of a king"—a recurrence of bubonic plague that was closing the Elizabethan theaters for months at a stretch, just as the coronavirus pandemic keeps closing our theaters now. Nonetheless, Shakespeare devoted very few words to any pestilence, even while the Black Death was ravaging his world. He turned away from the mind-numbing death counts that foster despair—the kind of statistics that we have come to know too well. The Bard preferred to imbue every death on his stage with some form of meaning.

Right now, many of us are seeking some form of meaning in the conflagration of disease and death that we are calling "the coronavirus pandemic." Most people alive today have never seen Pestilence burn through the world at this rate. The scope, speed, and complexity of this disease, and the dynamics it is revealing in our species at this time, are surpassing our ability to comprehend them. Medical scientists are offering us a kaleidoscopic view of the virus and its effects. Political pundits are expounding on its social impacts. Psychologists are reflecting on the inner turmoils that the pandemic is causing. And artists are attempting to see meaning in the mayhem and share what they see through their art. Each has described some of the pandemic's trees, but none have yet been able to compass its vast and deadly forest. We probably need a story for that.

In the opinion of many historians, storytelling is the most ancient form of human art. A strong story places our experience in a container of narrative, which enables us to consider our lives in a smaller and safer context, but also with a larger frame of reference. Stories give us perspective on our experience, factually and emotionally, which is why they have been our portals to personal meaning for millennia—well beyond recorded history. This has made of stories a kind of sustenance for the human soul. To quote the author Barry Lopez, "Sometimes a person needs a story more than food to stay alive."[1]

So it seems likely that if we want to discover some meaning in the

1. Lopez, Barry. *Crow and Weasel.* New York: Farrar Straus Giroux, 1990, p. 117

coronavirus pandemic, we should examine the fundamental story that carries its essence. What are the historical and contemporary settings of this story? Who are its characters? What is the narrative of this monumental event? And what might its meaningful consequences eventually be in our lives and our world?

My goal in this book is to discover that story—those settings and characters, that rough narrative, and those possible consequences. I will try to include the contributions of medical and social science whenever I can. But this will be more a work of storytelling than history. Let's see if we can identify the essential story of the coronavirus pandemic in comparison to its predecessors, and then discover some meaning in that story, at least enough meaning to keep our hearts and souls alive until we reach its conclusion.

The big questions are really the only ones worth considering, and colossal nerve has always been a prerequisite for such consideration.

– Alfred W. Crosby [2]

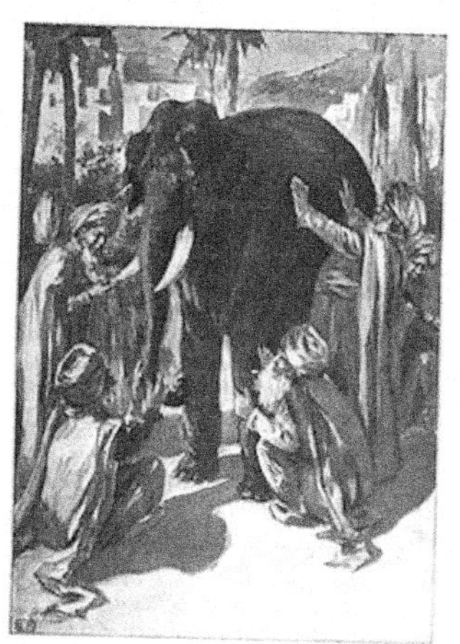

(Shutterstock)

The lore of ancient India describes an encounter between seven men and an elephant. Each man describes the elephant differently, depending on the body part he is touching. The leg is a "tree trunk," the flank is a "wall," the tusk is a "spear," the tail is a "rope." As they stand around the animal, each man carefully describes what he touches, but none of the men is comprehending "elephant."

In the original tale, all of the men's descriptions are incomplete, and therefore incorrect, because the men are blind. But when we live out this parable in real life, we don't draw incomplete conclusions because we are blind. We draw them because we are trying to describe a phenomenon so vast and complicated that it exceeds the scope of our individual comprehension. To paraphrase the cognitive scientist Emerson Pugh, "If life were so simple that we could understand it, we would be so simple that we couldn't."[3] We understand

2. Crosby, Alfred W. *The Columbian Exchange: Biological and Cultural Consequences of 1492.* Westport, CT: Greenwood, 2003, p. 177.

3. Pugh, George E. *The Biological Origin of Human Values* (Chapter 7: Mysteries of the

the chunk of a phenomenon that we can grasp with our limited human capacities, but we rarely grasp the total phenomenon.

This is why many of humanity's most important events have only been comprehended by people who have considered them from a distance—a further shore of elapsed time, remote geography, or distant expertise. Consider the fact that the actual story of the 1918 influenza pandemic was not fully comprehended, nor publicly described, until half a century after the pandemic's onset. That story was researched and written by a brilliant young historian named Alfred W. Crosby, who tripped over its catastrophic truth while he was researching an entirely different topic.[4]

Crosby went on to write a series of books that addressed massively pivotal events in human history, often from a scientific perspective, although Crosby himself was a historian. Crosby claimed that he was only able to grasp these stories because he was far enough removed from their events and subject matter to comprehend their scope and meaning. Of course, Crosby also possessed sweeping intelligence and stellar insight. But then, so did a lot of the people who lived through the events that Crosby described. And yet, they were never able to comprehend those events as he did.

Our world is currently in the throes of another massively pivotal event—a global pandemic the likes of which we have not seen since 1918, nor possibly even before that (depending on how this all turns out). Countless experts are working bravely, tirelessly, and creatively to solve the mystery of the novel coronavirus and its lethal offspring, Covid-19. I stand in awe of what they are trying to accomplish in their efforts to heal humanity and expand our understanding of Nature's mysteries.

However, as I read each piece of news about the coronavirus pandemic, and as I contemplate the intricate puzzle that these researchers are attempting to solve, I find myself thinking about the parable of the elephant. I wonder whether it might be possible to derive a more comprehensive sense of what this beast might be—this beast of a virus and this beast of a story. If the elephant parable is apt, it will require someone standing on a very distant shore, someone who can view the puzzle and its pieces from a more remote perspective, in order to get a sense of the elephant beyond its innumerable parts.

The whole is made up of its parts, of course, but the essence and story of elephant is something much larger than the sum of its parts. And it is

Mind, epigraph and footnote, p. 154). New York: Basic Books, 1977. The original Emerson Pugh quote is, "If the mind were so simple that we could understand it, we would be so simple that we couldn't."

4. Crosby, Alfred W. *Epidemic and Peace, 1918.* Westport, CT: Greenwood Press, 1976.

the elephant in the story of every pandemic—that is, the pandemic's larger context and essence—that gives us a sense of meaning for the suffering that the pandemic entails. This is why we cherish stories, and even depend upon them for our survival, as Barry Lopez so wisely observed.

But how can we possibly frame the gargantuan story of the coronavirus and Covid-19?

Well, let's start with the fact that each of humanity's famous pandemics is really a unique drama. Each is like a stage play that begins with a specific context of time and place—a vast set onto which the disease takes its first steps. And the disease itself, as the invader-protagonist of the play, has a specific personality. Similarly, we have two sets of characters who defend against the disease: 1) the biological defenders of the human immune system which fight ferociously against the pathogen, and 2) the defending behaviors of the human beings who are under pandemic invasion.

Today, we can read some of the stories left to us by people who suffered in the historical pandemics—both the people who perished in their ghastly onslaughts and the people who survived them, with scars on their bodies and souls. And at the end of each story, after the disease-invader has left the stage, we see a new setting—the world that the disease leaves behind. That world is part of the story, too. Each pandemic leaves its marks upon the world—marks that are excruciating, but not entirely negative, despite the mass graves and unspeakable suffering. This gift of a larger view on terrible tragedy is one reason the ancient Greeks considered theater a healing art—because even the theater's most horrific stories offer the redemption of larger context and deeper meaning.

My goal in writing this book is to see how much of the coronavirus "drama" I can place upon this metaphorical stage. Will I succeed? One reason for optimism is that I am regarding these awful stories from several kinds of distance, as Alfred Crosby regarded the subjects he described. I am not living in a place that is terribly afflicted by the virus. I am not a healthcare worker overwhelmed by the needs of Covid-19 patients. I am neither an immunologist, nor an epidemiologist, nor a bio-historian, all of whom would be experts on the vast forest of information pertaining to these events, but whose expertise would force them to focus on the details of its countless trees.[5]

In addition to my distant perspective, my special advantages are 1) a talent for pattern recognition, and 2) a knack for invoking metaphors

5. That being said, I do have knack for finding key research that pertains to the topics that interest me. And I believe that whatever information I choose to share should be made *easily* accessible to those with whom I share it. That is the reason there is no gigantic bibliography at the end of this book. With the exception of some very specific resources that appear as footnotes located directly below where their information is cited, everything you will read here is available to anyone who possesses curiosity and an access to Wikipedia.

that can draw useful meanings from the patterns I detect. In my work as a practitioner of Jungian psychology, I help my clients look for patterns in their dreams, and I support them as they describe the meanings they sense beneath those patterns, often through metaphorical connections. That task applies to nighttime dreams, but it also applies to the "dreams" of body symptoms, individual life events, and the collective patterns of world events. In truth, I perceive most of life through the lens of metaphor.

It was the opinion of Carl Jung that metaphor serves as the winged workhorse of the human psyche. Metaphor lifts us back and forth between the understandable and the incomprehensible. That is why we can see how the elephant parable is relevant to the task of describing this pandemic; it performs the literal Greek meaning of the word metaphor (μεταφέρω)—"to transport over." It transports us from the familiar to the fantastic, and sometimes beyond—to what was previously unimaginable. Best of all, metaphor preserves the complexity of the mysterious thing, even as it makes it accessible to us. Metaphor is my native tongue, and it is the primary language I will use to tell this pandemic story.

Yes, I do wish that Alfred Crosby were alive to untangle this tale and solve its puzzle, because he would do it brilliantly. But Professor Crosby entered a drama beyond life in 2018, leaving behind his books as the stars by which we must navigate a narrative as vast and treacherous as this one. I write this book partly in tribute to Professor Crosby's unique genius, hoping that whatever it achieves will do him honor, and that its failings will be assigned entirely to myself. But more than that, I hope that my search for meaning in the harrowing land of pandemic disease will honor the uncountable multitudes of people who have lost to Pestilence everything they held most dear, including their lives, their loved ones, and all sense of meaning and hope. And perhaps this book can also provide some encouragement to modern people who feel they are losing those same things today.

Let us begin…

CHAPTER 1

This is How Pandemic Stories Begin...

(Shutterstock)

And so from hour to hour we ripe and ripe,
And then from hour to hour we rot and rot;
And thereby hangs a tale.

– William Shakespeare,
As You Like It, II.vii

Those who cannot remember the past
are condemned to repeat it.

– George Santayana[6]

Every story begins somewhere, and sometime, with certain events and certain people. It is rarely clear which comes first—the time, the place, the events, or the people. So let's just begin this story with one of its central characters.

He was a man who was the leader of his formidable country. Mind you, one would never have guessed, based on his abrasive nature and the tawdry events of his earlier life, that he would have achieved the position of power that he held by the time this story began. You see, by the time this story began, this man had quite probably become the most powerful

6. Santayana, George. *Life of Reason or The Phases of Human Progress, One Volume Edition.* New York: Charles Scribner's Sons, 1955.

person in the world.

He was not, in the opinion of most people, a very likeable man. He was ruthless, self-absorbed, cunning, and untrustworthy. Nonetheless, despite his repellent traits, the man seemed to have a genius for accumulating power and persuading others to do his bidding. Perhaps it was because he knew how to appeal to the lowest of human motivations—greed, fear, and the desire to be better than someone else.

It is uncertain what the man's own motivations were for himself. Wealth was certainly important to him, and he had amassed a considerable amount of that. But he was driven far beyond the accumulation of wealth, so he clearly wasn't content with mere affluence.

And he burned through women like a wildfire torching prairie grass, ravaging all the women who caught his eye and came within his grasp. But it seemed that he had no real liking for women; he devoured them only as fuel for his insatiable hunger.

That said, the man did eventually settle upon one woman, a famous beauty whose ambitions were a match for his own. She had been born into obscurity and privation, but she had advanced herself through the world of sexual commerce. And that was where she had attracted the man's attention. Clearly, she was more than a skilled and beautiful prostitute. There must have been something about her that the man recognized as similar to himself. Eventually, he chose this sex worker as the wife with whom he would remain longer than any other woman. In fact, she became his wife and his partner in conquest.

Yes, it seems that among his considerable appetites, conquest and power were the hungers that drove this man most relentlessly. In spite of the diverse nature of the realm he acquired when he became a leader, the man was determined to consolidate its far-flung riches and myriad benefits under his singular hand. He pursued a form of centralized nationalism that had previously been thought obsolete. But there was something about the ferocious drive of this man that resurrected the old despotic forms and rendered them as a new world order under his rule. Perhaps it was because the man's totalitarian goals seemed to promise his populace some security and renewed dominance in a world that felt to them chaotic and decomposing.

The man was well on his way to accomplishing so much of what he wanted. He had consolidated the power of his realm, manipulated its established governance, and exploited its resources to his own ends. It was all just within his reach. And then...

There came rumors of a disease that was brewing in a far country across the sea—a country that was a partner in trade with the country of this power-hungry man, though it was distant in its geography and cultural norms.

At first, the rumors were vague and, possibly, not even true. Certainly, the man himself dismissed them as trivial...the inconsequential or malicious fabrications of his enemies. He marched forward with his plans of unifying his constituents, banishing his foes, and converting his nation into the centralized empire of his desires. Even when the rumors of contagion proved to be based in actual records of malady and death, both of which were creeping closer to his lands, the man pursued his goals of conquest and consolidation as if he could conquer the disease in the same way he had conquered all of his other opponents. That is, what could not be bought off could be bullied or bludgeoned into submission. Or it could simply be ignored until it begged for mercy or departed in despair.

Eventually, the disease reached the man's own shores, his own cities, his own peoples. Suddenly, it became clear that everything this man had hoped to achieve, everything he had hoped to conquer, everything he had hoped to consolidate under his iron hand was slipping from his grasp. Disease and death were jeopardizing everything he had felt was owed to him. His shock, outrage, and furious attempts to prevail were for naught. Pestilence was a foe that fought on principles this man did not comprehend. Pestilence employed methods that he could not counter or defeat. The man was nearly mad with the thought that he could be brought so low by something so invisible and implacable...

This is *not* the story of the coronavirus pandemic in America. The man in this story is *not* Donald Trump, and his wife is not Melania. The date of this story is 541 CE and the man is the Emperor Justinian, the tyrant of Constantinople who, with his prostitute wife Theodora, attempted to reunite and reign supreme over the realm that had previously been known as the Roman Empire. On the brink of achieving this massive conquest, Justinian's world burst into bacterial flame with the pandemic that came to carry his name—"The Plague of Justinian." This world conqueror, who conceived and nearly created a second Roman Empire through a mind-bending campaign of violence, manipulation, and tyranny, met his nemesis in the microscopic bacillus we now call *yersinia pestis*...plague.

Okay, let's try this again...

Allow me to introduce you to a group of men—oligarchs, to speak plainly—who wielded nearly everything that counted as power in their portion of the world. These oligarchs didn't possess *all* the political power there was to wield. But they officially wielded enough overt power, and they quietly manipulated enough covert power, so that they pretty much ran whatever was worth running in their portion of the globe.

Similarly, these oligarchs didn't possess *all* the wealth of their world, but they possessed a great deal of the world's wealth. And beyond that, they controlled many of the banking and commercial enterprises that juggled the rest of their world's assets.

Most important of all, perhaps, was that these men had instilled in a majority of their people the unshakeable conviction that the values and beliefs of their society were superior to all others—an ethos of exceptionalism in which theirs was the most enviable social system available to humankind. By means of their persuasions and promises (as well as their threats), these men had convinced most of the people in their world that their way was the *best* way, and perhaps the *only* way, to live safely and happily, and that any other way of living was of dubious merit, to the point of being evil. In other words, these oligarchs had convinced their people that God was on *their* side...and no one else's.

When a group of people holds as much power as these oligarchs, when they essentially make it a habit to play God, it is easy for them to believe that they actually *are* gods...or at least, god-like. So when word came to these men about a disease that was afflicting a country far removed from theirs in distance and beliefs, they dismissed it as a fitting punishment for that country's heathen ways. They believed that their more exalted way of being, their God-blessed conduct, would protect them from the foreign affliction.

Then, when that foreign disease had the temerity to arrive on *their* shores, they relied on their belief in their godlike powers to protect them from the alien nuisance. They gathered in their sacred places, fortified by the riches of their plunder and the esteemed icons of their power, and they exercised what they believed to be their superior authority over this immigrant invader.

The immigrant invader was not impressed. Disease and death ravaged the land of the oligarchs. It decimated their constituents physically, but even more disastrously for the oligarchs, it eventually made their loyal believers doubt what they had been told and believed for many years. It slowly occurred to the people that perhaps their leaders were not as God-blessed as they had claimed they were...as even the leaders themselves may have believed they were. By the tens, hundreds, and even thousands, people fell away from the oligarchy, as they fell into their sickbeds and, often, into their graves.

This, too, is *not* the story of the coronavirus pandemic in America. These oligarchs are *not* the conservative evangelists of the Republican party. The date is 1347, and the oligarchy in this story is the Roman Catholic Church. In the early 14th century, the power of the Catholic Church was absolute and unchallenged throughout Europe. No aspect of medieval European life was independent of the Church's dictate and judgment. Power, money, and influence were wielded in equal measure by the Church fathers, on levels both massive and mundane. But most importantly, the Church controlled the hearts, minds, and souls of medieval Europeans. Until this point.

As omnipotent as the Church seemed to be, its leaders and followers were eventually forced to accept that Christianity was not as powerful as the same terrifying force—invisible in its form, but unmistakable in its effects—that had set fire to the dreams of Emperor Justinian. Once again, a group of humans who had stood unconquered in the world were brought to their knees by the microscopic might of *yersinia pestis*...plague.

Now, shall we have another go at this?

It was a splendid land, as rich in its human resources as in its natural resources. Although the land was occupied by people of diverse ethnicities, they were a magnificent people when taken as a whole—abundant in their cultural wealth, brilliant in their sciences, artistically gifted, and spiritually devout in myriad ways. Sometimes these diverse groups lived in relative harmony, but frequently, their differing cultures brought them to bloody violence. Still, they had cohabited on this beautiful land for many, many years, and they mostly held an equilibrium with each other, in between their eruptions of dispute. Their world view was based on the continuity of their lives over the time they had coexisted upon their land, and although there was smoldering conflict, these peoples had survived it all by dint of their hard work, strong beliefs, robust constitutions, and a conviction that they were the most fortunate and God-blessed people in the world.

When a new disease arrived from foreign soil, it erupted among these people almost before they knew what was happening. Their prodigious intellects were sabotaged by their conflicts with each other (and, yes, by their arrogance, too), and their resourcefulness was neutralized by their inexperience with their foe. This was an alien invader, transported from across the sea by people that most of the victims would never see. Indeed, even those who initially transported the invader were unaware of what they had carried to this land—disease and death beyond anything they could comprehend in their state of ocean-hopping privilege. Their own ignorance and arrogance on this matter were equal to those of the peoples they were infecting.

In the end, the inhabitants of this beautiful land—no matter their culture, religion, or location in the landscape—were felled like mown wheat by the ruthless blade of the primary invading pathogen and its companion afflictions. The inhabitants of the land discovered that the only dispute that mattered wasn't with each other, nor even with foreigners from outside their country. The only war that mattered was with *disease*, disease beyond anything they had ever encountered...

As you might have guessed by now, this is another story that is *not* the story of the coronavirus pandemic in America, although we are finally on the correct continent. But the people in this story are *not* the diverse ethnic and racial groups of the United States. The date is 1493, and these are the original "Americans," the peoples who inhabited the New World for thousands of years before the Europeans arrived. The original peoples of the New World were brilliant, ferocious, proud, and accomplished. Some were stronger, richer, and fiercer than others, but they were all equal when they faced the pestilential enemy that cut them down, nation after nation. It was really a troupe of diseases that ravaged the post-Columbian New World, but the brutal leader of that deadly brigade was the ancient virus that we have come to call *variola major*...smallpox.

Okay, just one more try...

Of the many sufferings that can torment humankind, the afflictions of Famine and Disease are equaled in their cruelty only by those of War. And as we all know, war does not always involve literal weapons and explicit death. There are wars of finance, wars of influence, and wars of psychological manipulation that can claim as many lives as wars that involve blood and armaments.

In this story, we meet two world powers who are at war, the majority of which has been waged for years without a single shot being fired. Acts of financial and diplomatic aggression have been committed, and endless volleys of deadly words have been exchanged. The poisonous tactics of trade embargoes and sneaky deals have inflicted casualties on both sides. And through it all, the brutality of their combat has been disguised by ruthless negotiating and verbal flimflammery.

When disease erupted in the midst of this war, neither side wanted to acknowledge its seriousness. Epithets and blaming were exchanged, and rampant accusations were fired back and forth as the contagion expanded. There was a desire by both parties to hide the severity of the problem, mostly so that both could carry on with the business of their aggressive competition. Even when it became clear that the contagion had broken beyond their control, both sides engaged in dissembling, denial, and magical thinking in a vain attempt to sweep the problem under the rug that they shared with the entire world...along with the pandemic that was now raging unabated.

As a result, the disease roared around the world, infecting a sizeable majority of the human species and killing an unconscionable number of those who were infected...the innocent victims of a war for global dominance between two power-mad nations.

And yet again, this is *not* the story of the coronavirus pandemic. The date is 1918, and the two warring nations are *not* the United States and China, but rather, the United States and Germany. Both countries were burdened with leaders and constituents who have been described as "stark raving patriotic,"[7] and their nationalist madness drove decisions that poured gas on the fire of their incendiary pandemic. It was a pandemic that became a global disaster. Several current world leaders have referred to the novel coronavirus as "just the flu." But it was, in fact, "just the flu" that incinerated the world during and after World War I—a version of flu that scientists now call *influenzavirus A, type H1N1*, but that most of us know as "the 1918 flu."

♦ ♦ ♦

Whenever we find ourselves in the middle of a crisis, especially a crisis of global proportions, it is our healthy nature to ask, "How could this possibly have happened?" In the midst of mayhem, we try to detect any patterns of context and causation that can give us a handle on the chaos.

Context and causation are the gifts offered to us by historians, and also by storytellers with historical vision. To paraphrase the philosopher George Santayana, if we want to avoid repeating the past, we must learn what it can teach us. To that great truth can be added the fact that learning from the past allows us to place the present in a larger context, a context where we can perceive it with greater insight. Then, if we are clever and fortunate, we can step carefully toward a future that is better than the one where denial and ignorance will otherwise dump us.

In the four pandemic origin stories I have told, we have encountered the contributing elements of 1) a power-hungry leader whose priorities

7. Crosby, Alfred W. *America's Forgotten Pandemic: The Influenza of 1918.* Cambridge, UK.: Cambridge University Press, 1976/1989, p. 46

and tactics rendered him incapable of effective response to the threat that eventually consumed his populace and demolished his ambitions, 2) a power-obsessed oligarchy whose inflated "god complex" led them to convince their people that the threat of disease could be defeated with blind faith and loyal conduct, 3) an assembly of diverse and disputing cultures whose varied beliefs and history of harms, along with their inexperience at being global victims, led them to set a world record for disease and death, and 4) a pair of power-mad nations whose rivalry for global dominance possibly unleashed, and certainly augmented, the lethal force of a viral beast that preyed upon the world...including themselves.

It should be easy to recognize all four of these catalytic factors in the story of the coronavirus pandemic in America. But to these specific catalysts, we can also add the elements that are common to nearly *all* stories of pandemic disease, no matter the species, the pathogen, the location, or the historical moment. These facilitators of contagion can be considered the basic ingredients for igniting and fueling an epidemic blaze, so let's take a closer look at them.

An epidemic is like a forest fire.
The earlier you get there, before the flames are rampant,
the better off you will do.
And that is especially true of long incubation diseases,
where the smoldering damage has spread a lot more than
you realize by the time you see the smoke.

– Don Francis, M.D., Epidemiologist specializing in HIV/AIDS and Ebola[8]

#1—Population density and interconnectedness

In all four of the pandemic stories I have told, the afflicted populations had achieved sufficient density and interconnection to sustain the contagion. To borrow from Dr. Francis's metaphor above, it's just like the tree densities and connective ladder fuels that sustain massive forest fires; the combustible materials must be present in great enough density and proximity or the fire will burn out for lack of fuel. Thus, dense populations that are interconnected allow the disease invader to find new hosts to colonize and consume before it burns through all of its current hosts.

This notion of diseases being like fires is the basis for the recent computer modeling for epidemic predictions. In the last decade, formulae have been

8. PBS *Frontline,* December 2, 2004 https://www.pbs.org/wgbh/pages/frontline/aids/interviews/francis.html.

developed that calculate the minimum population necessary to ignite and sustain an epidemic for any given disease. Technically, four key factors in a population contribute to a pandemic's ignition (which is called the "outbreak threshold" or T_O) and contagiousness (which is called "reproductive ratio" or R_O).[9] Simply stated, all pandemics require a population that is numerous enough, with clusters of people that are close enough together, so that it will sustain the disease while it expands its colonization to new human populations. The fire of the epidemic will burn out if:

1. The disease is not contagious enough;
2. There are too few people in the population;
3. The people in the population are too widely spaced;
4. The disease kills off too many people before it can infect new people.

But with rapid enough contagion, dense enough population, groups of people spaced closely enough together, and a low enough kill ratio, an epidemic can last for a *very* long time. In fact, depending on its mode of transmission, an epidemic can last for *centuries.*

This, in fact, is exactly what the plague did after arriving in Europe in 1347. Even when Shakespeare was writing in 1600, the theaters were frequently shut down because of plague outbreaks. And yes, *it was exactly the same plague that had landed in Europe 250 years prior.* It's really just a matter of arithmetic. Pandemic diseases only require a sufficient number of people, gathered in close enough groups, with no anti-contagion protocols or vaccines, and a low enough kill ratio to leave enough survivors. That's all a pandemic needs to persist...even for centuries.

Forget "herd immunity." Without the artificially-induced herd immunity of a vaccine, effective herd immunity takes *millennia* to develop. And with the deadlier diseases, it never develops at all. Those diseases kill us too effectively to permit the procreation of immune offspring. Consider plague, smallpox, measles, chicken pox, or any of the other endemic diseases that have killed (and can still kill) millions of people, thousands of years after they first colonized human bodies. Natural herd immunity is a tantalizing but treacherous delusion born of desperate optimism and narcissistic denial.

Returning to the realities of pandemic contagion, let's first look at the role of population density and interconnectedness in the four major pandemics of human history:

9. Hartfield, Matthew and Samuel Alizon. "Introducing the Outbreak Threshold in Epidemiology." *PLoS Pathogens*, May 2022. https://paperity.org/p/61068334/introducing-the-outbreak-threshold-in-epidemiology.

Plague of Justinian (541 CE) The expansion of the Roman Empire, even in its decline, had improved the safety of life and travel so much that, compared to prior époques, humans could procreate and migrate with ease throughout Europe, the Mediterranean, and the Middle East. And so could the rats who depended upon human settlements. And so could the fleas who were carried by the rats. And so could the *yersinia pestis* that infected them all.

Black Death (1347 CE) The same was true by the mid-14th century CE. The rising level of social structure and security, after recovering from the fall of the second Roman Empire in the 6th century, had allowed human population levels and commerce routes to return to early Roman states of prosperity. Once again, humans, rats, fleas, and plague could proliferate and travel freely across the land and seas. And so they all did.

Post-Columbian Plural Pandemic (1493-1600 CE) Although the nations of the pre-Columbian New World had not mastered ocean travel, they were *very* adept at land travel. And although their nations were independent and often in conflict, they were not at war *constantly*, which allowed them to enjoy a web of commerce and communication along established travel routes. In addition, the abundant resources in the New World permitted rapid population growth, even to the point where overpopulation was occasionally a problem for one nation or another. Thus, for the most part, the New World nations represented an interconnected system of thriving population centers by the time the Old World sailors and their pathogens made landfall in 1492. In terms of the forest fire metaphor, the New World provided lots of human fuel and a perfect network of fuel sources for the following Old World diseases to thrive, ***in addition to smallpox***:

Plague
Measles
Typhus
Cholera
Scarlet fever
Influenza

Diphtheria
Chicken pox
Whooping cough
Yellow fever
Malaria

Most deadly of all, however, was the fact that the New World inhabitants lacked the inbred advantage of the Spaniards who, like all Old World inhabitants, had lived closely with animals for millennia. That is, the Spanish invaders were the descendants of humans who had survived the diseases they had acquired from the animals they had husbanded for thousands of years. Although a huge number of Old World children and adults still died from those diseases (their "herd" was *not* immune), the partial resistance they had developed over thousands of years allowed a sufficient number of their population to survive their childhood disease parade, as we currently do. Thus, the Spaniards had become carriers of these diseases, serving as containers of a cargo that was repeatedly lethal to the biologically "naïve" population of the Americas—people who had no immunity whatsoever to *any* of these diseases.[10]

1918 Influenza (1918-20 CE) If we can say that the population levels of the lands afflicted in 541, 1347, and 1493 were robust enough to support a pandemic, then it would be fair to say that by 1918, human procreativity had produced a crop of human hosts that could satisfy even the most voracious invader. Consider this comparative chart of the world's population over these centuries:

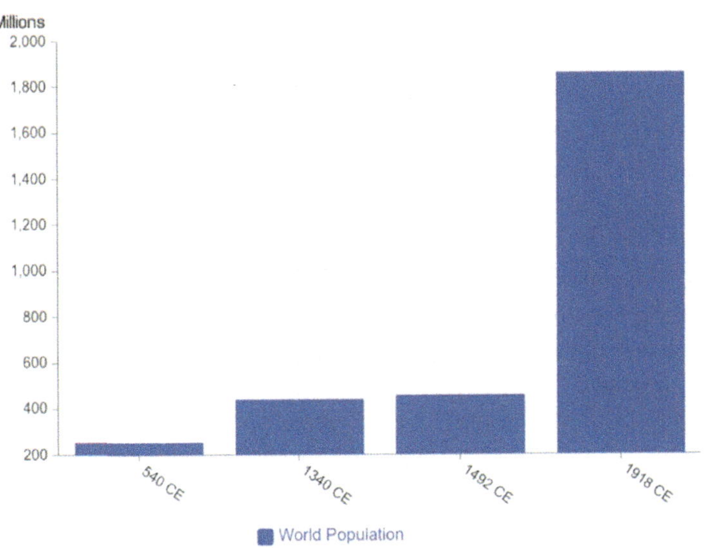

10. To answer a question that you might reasonably be asking right now, there was only one documented disease that was previously unknown in the Old World, and that the Columbians and other *conquistadors* brought back to Europe. That disease was *syphilis*. In a miniscule compensation for the biological disaster that befell the New World, the Old World inhabitants were as vulnerable to syphilis as the New World inhabitants were to all the Old World diseases. So when syphilis first came to the Old World, it was a ravaging disease—highly contagious, brutal in its effects, and often quickly lethal. Moreover, syphilis was sexually transmitted, so it had the effect of eroding Old World social structures, as it shattered the false assumptions of marital fidelity in 15th and 16th century Europe. Certainly, this was not equal to the disaster that befell the New World, but it was nonetheless a small biological vengeance. Tragically, of course, none of the New World pandemic victims ever heard about it.

Given the advent of ocean travel for masses of people by 1918, added to the invention of the locomotive and the expansion of rail travel, plus the mushrooming population of the world, it is clear that by the time *influenza Type A, H1N1* made land on human soil in March 1918, there was a vast resource of human fuel that was easily accessible for it to consume—some to merely infect, and some to annihilate.

And remember, once again, that the most successful diseases do *not* kill a majority of their hosts. If they did, the pandemic would burn out before the disease could spread to new hosts. The 1918 flu only killed approximately 3% of those it infected...which still produced, by modern estimates, a death toll of between 50 to 100 million hosting humans. That would be between 400 and 900 million people in today's global population, or between one and three times the current U.S. population.

#2—Stressors in the physical and societal environment

Although high population density imposes its own kind of stress on the people who live in such circumstances, there are environmental factors that have even greater impact on human existence than population density. Consider the fact that years of drought can place *any* forest on the brink of devastation when it stands before an approaching fire. The same is true of human populations that stand before an invading pathogen. Environmental adversities and social stressors weaken a human population and give the disease a greater advantage for contagion and mortality. Let's take a look at how this factor influenced the historical pandemics:

Plague of Justinian (541 CE) During the decades prior to the plague, the violent campaign of consolidation that Justinian inflicted on his realm was a terrible stressor for its inhabitants, independent of their population densities and environmental challenges. In addition, we now know that a massive pyroclastic blast, probably originating around 539 from the now-collapsed Ilopango volcano in El Salvador, created a "volcanic winter" that lasted for years, causing global cooling throughout Europe and Asia. Added to the food shortages that the population suffered during these cold years, the subsequent migrations of humans and animals out of Mongolia and into southern lands would have brought with them the vermin of central Asia, including the Oriental rat flea, which has always been the favored mode of transport for the plague bacillus.

Black Death (1347 CE) The population of Europe had already been weakened by the start of the Hundred Years War (1337-1453), which ignited widespread civil disorder, the destruction of livelihoods, and chronic famine throughout the continent. But more than that, much of the world was in the throes of what is now called "the Little Ice Age," beginning around the start of the 14th century. Crops failed and famine was rampant, especially in the years from 1315-1317. The population was thus greatly weakened by starvation and cold weather, which continued for several decades. This period of cold was either initiated or exacerbated by several major volcanic events in the late 1200s century. None were as large as the Ilopango pyroclasm in the 6th century, but the sum of these volcanic events combined to produce or augment the perpetual cold winter of this period. Once again, the humans and vermin of the Mongolian steppes moved south, along with their perennial companions, the plague-bearing fleas, and the human population in Europe was defenseless in its weakened condition.

Post-Columbian Plural Pandemic (1493-1600 CE) In the New World of the 15th century, there was no presiding organization or unifying system among the myriad nations that were widely dispersed in distance and culture. As a result, there was no ability to prepare for or combat the incomprehensible barrage of diseases that pummeled most of the New World inhabitants as there had been, at least to a minimal degree, in 6th and 14th century Europe. True, there had been no means of rapid communication in ancient or medieval Europe to spread word of their devastating plague pandemics. But the nations of those worlds were, at least, undergoing some form of unification—Justinian in the first case, and Roman Catholic in the second. As we saw from the earlier description of Justinian's denial and the Church's arrogance, no immediate use was made of leadership in combatting these contagions, but some protocols of control were finally instituted. (For example, the word "quarantine" originated in the Italian word "quaranta" or "forty" referring to the forty days that foreign boats and caravans had to sequester plague-free before they were allowed into an Italian city during the Black Death.)

By contrast, when European invaders set foot on the interior lands of the New World after 1600, they often found territories that were nearly devoid of human inhabitants. They assumed that the lands had always been that way, because they had no way of knowing that *between 85 and 95% of the 100 million indigenous residents of the New World's had died between 1492 and 1600.* The great distances of space and time in that tragic story had swallowed the terrible truth of what has been called "possibly the greatest demographic disaster in the history of the world."[11] During the 16th century, the New World inhabitants succumbed to inferno after inferno of humanity's most dreadful diseases, led by the scourge of smallpox. It would be like burning down one forest multiple times in less than a hundred years. Nothing would be left but cold ash.

1918 Influenza (1918-20 CE) Although the environmental conditions in the world of 1918 were not particularly adverse, the morbidity and mortality levels of the 1918 flu were magnified exponentially by several horrific elements in the physical and societal environment of World War I:

1. Massive troop movements around the world spread the disease widely in ways that would not otherwise have occurred.
2. Soldiers on *all* sides suffered unspeakably foul conditions, both in the trenches and in the barracks, which made perfect breeding grounds for epidemic infection.
3. The Germans deployed the chemical agent "mustard gas" (dichlorethyl sulfide), which blistered the throat and lungs and left any survivors extremely vulnerable to respiratory infection. The gas affected the German soldiers as well as the Allied soldiers, leaving them all with severe respiratory vulnerabilities.
4. Any efforts at isolation, quarantine, and social distancing for troops and civilians were resisted or rescinded by the combatant governments so that war production could proceed apace. The conditions in the war materiel factories especially augmented contagion, as did conditions in the troop barracks and transports.
5. All news of the epidemic was minimized or suppressed on both sides in the war, so that losses would not be recognized...neither by the enemy nor by supporters on the home front. In the absence of global news services, it was possible for people to believe that the flu was only affecting their local communities, without ever recognizing its widespread devastation. The lack of general public awareness of the flu's destruction contributed to the public's lack of effective response, including demands for anti-contagion action by the government.

This summary strongly suggests that, in addition to the disturbing social coincidences between the four historical pandemics and the coronavirus

11. Denevan, William M. *The Native Population of the Americas in 1492.* University of Wisconsin Press, 1992. *Project MUSE* muse.jhu.edu/book/8750

pandemic in America, we can add these factors from the four historical pandemics to our own now:

Population density, interconnectedness, and environmental stressors in 2020 CE

If the population densities during prior pandemics offered human fuel that was simply sufficient to ignite a conflagration of contagion, the levels of human fuel in our world are *astoundingly* well-suited to the needs of a hungry disease. Consider, for example, the population densities of the world in the prior four pandemics, as compared to the world's population today:

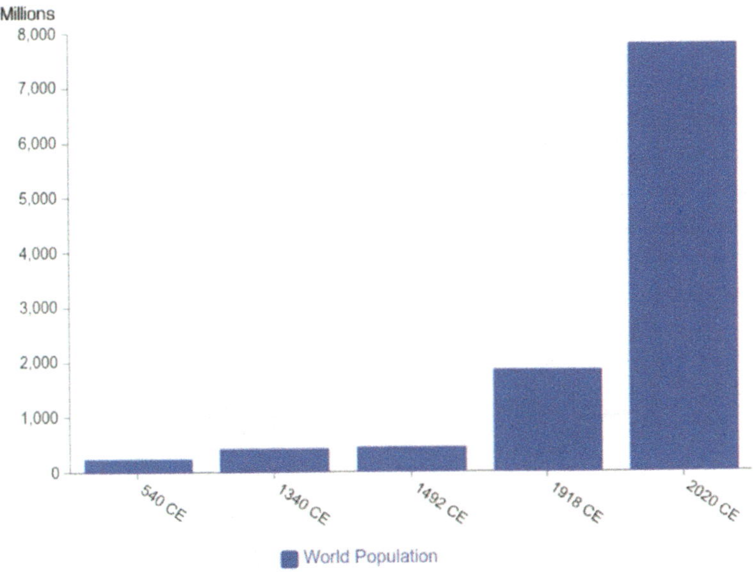

And not only is our population exponentially larger and denser than the populations of prior pandemic worlds, but the speed and ease of travel makes the contagion options super-charged for any modern pathogen. This is why the pandemics of the 6th, 14th, and 15th centuries required *years* to expand throughout their worlds. The 1918 pandemic required *months*. But the novel coronavirus pandemic only took a few *weeks* to encompass the globe.

The human beings of earlier pandemics lived with environmental adversities and social stressors that we can barely comprehend today. Their air, soil, and waters may have been less polluted than ours, but their conditions of hygiene and medical care were horrific by our standards. Moreover, they lived with situations of political instability and violence that America has only known during the Civil War. Nonetheless, our levels of population density, environmental contamination, and social discord are pervasive and destabilizing, even though they are much more subtle than the vermin, filth, and daily dangers that harrowed the humans of 6th and 14th century Europe. Let's consider one American city for examples of these elements, comparing its conditions as recently as 1950 with its conditions today.

Let me introduce you to the 1950s version of...Los Angeles.

The city of Los Angeles measures approximately 500 square miles. In other words, one could theoretically drive its perimeter in 90 minutes. In 1950, the population of Los Angeles was approximately 2 million people. In 2020, its population was more than 4 million people. In 1950, there were approximately 25 miles of freeway in the greater Los Angeles area. Today, there are over 500 miles of freeway in the same area.

A flight from Los Angeles to Tokyo lasted 32 hours in 1950, and only the most privileged people could afford to take it. Today, the same flight takes one third the amount of time and thousands can afford it...so they take it. Traveling between Los Angeles and Beijing took days or weeks in 1950. Today, it takes less than 20 hours.

Let's look at the Los Angeles of the 1950s and the Los Angeles of today:

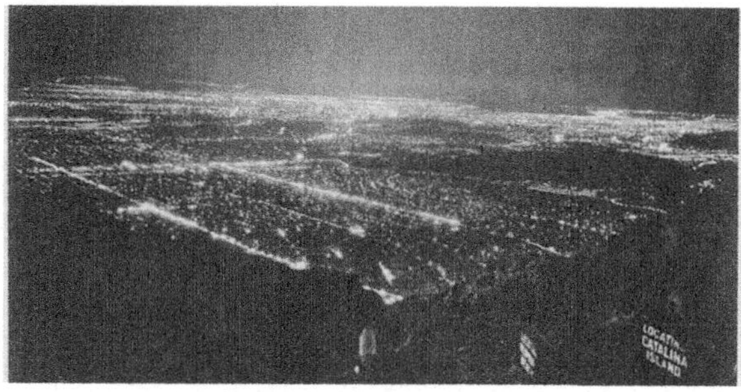

Los Angeles circa 1950 (Shutterstock)

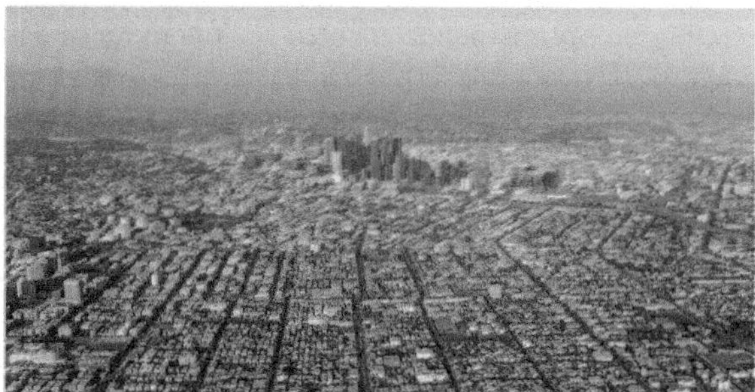

Los Angeles circa 2020 (Shutterstock)

The air quality of Los Angeles was already deplorable by 1950, but we have an idea of what it might have been before the arrival of human automotive transport, based upon what happened during the recent "lockdown" in the coronavirus pandemic. This brief reprieve from respiratory stress was not enough to protect Los Angelenos against the ravages of the coronavirus, but the comparative photos depict what damage their respiratory systems had already sustained when the virus arrived after years of smog.

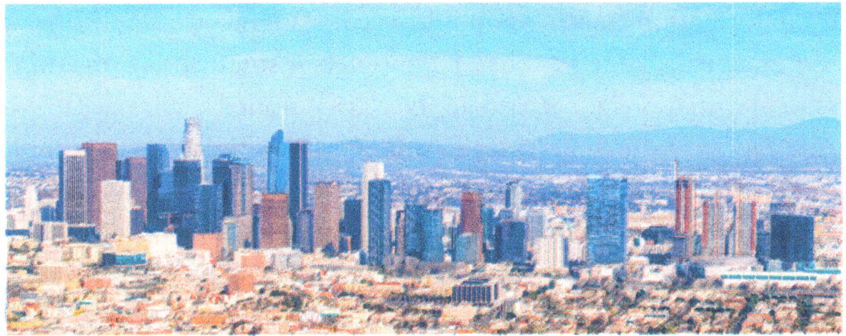

Los Angeles without air pollution (Shutterstock)

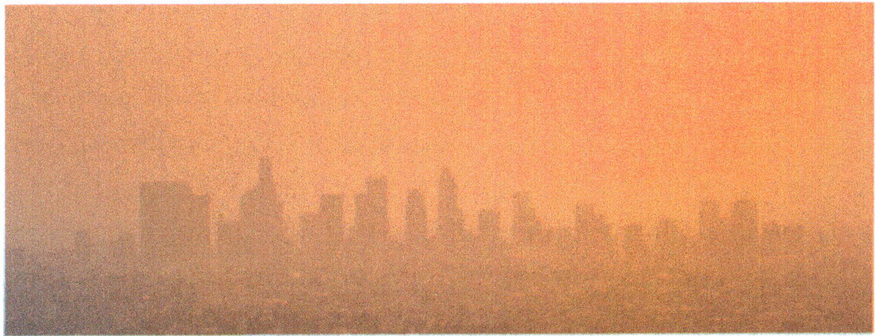

Los Angeles with air pollution (Shutterstock)

And what about the social stressors that we discussed earlier in the fueling of pandemic conflagrations?

Let's consider the fact that the major nations with the worst statistics in terms of control and recovery in the coronavirus pandemic were initially those with the three of the most totalitarian leaders at the beginning of the Covid pandemic—Russia, Brazil, and perhaps worst of all...the United States. In other words, if a country's leadership is intolerant of dissent, repressive toward opposition, and dismissive of information that counters its preferred narrative, the country is very unlikely, as one would predict, to muster the national unity and consensus that is required to combat a pandemic disease.

In addition, years of war led to a chaotic state in all of the historical pandemics stories I have recounted—Justinian's wars of conquest in the early 6th century, the Hundred Years' War in the early 14th century, the perpetual combat among the pre-Columbian American nations in the 15th century, and the stinking miasma of World War I in 1918. In 2020, the wars have been more metaphorical, but no less corrosive to the well-being of America's population. To name a few—the widening gap between our "haves" and "have-nots," the expanding ambitions of our multinational corporations, the exploitation of our natural and human resources to the benefit of a tiny minority, and the increasing loss of individual identity and potency as our population has soared.

Yes, information transmission is nearly instantaneous in our time, and it is available to anyone who has a computer or smartphone, making our access to information far better than the class-stratified snail's pace to which information was limited in historic pandemics. But information is not the same as knowledge and wisdom. We may be wallowing in some things that our ancestors would have cherished—better access to nutrition, education, health care, human rights, and most of all, infinite quantities of information. But sadly, we have lost ground in our access to authenticity, intimacy, contemplation, and *meaning*.

The end result today is a world population, and particularly an *American* population, that is better fed, better educated, better protected, and much healthier than in prior pandemics. But we are rendered sadly vulnerable by other stressors that did not torment our ancestors. We may know more, but we do not *understand* more about all that we know. Our inundation with information (including *mis*information and *dis*information), our entrancement with the latest loud and shiny object, and our addiction to speed in all responses have rendered us foolishly inept when it comes to making wise use of the resources at our disposal. As a consequence, the Covid statistics in America are chronically abysmal. Our foolishness and arrogance—the myth of American exceptionalism—have made us a menace to those whom we always believed were less privileged than we.

Thinking back to what we have learned about the ways in which population density and interconnectedness, along with environmental adversities, can accelerate the spread of pandemic disease, it becomes clear that even a privileged country like America and an especially privileged city like Los Angeles—home to movie stars and sports celebrities—can be the perfect candidate for colonization by an enterprising disease.

And so it has. By August 9, 2020, among the 4 million people in Los Angeles, 200,000 had been infected with novel coronavirus, and 5,000 of those people had died. By contrast, in the city of Kano, Nigeria (also home to 4 million inhabitants), 1,600 people had been infected with novel coronavirus and 54 had died. One could hardly call Nigeria a stress-free environment. Nonetheless, the statistics prove that it was not as welcoming to the novel coronavirus as was Los Angeles...or any other comparable American city.

♦ ♦ ♦

Taken together, the stories of humanity's four greatest pandemics suggest that the coronavirus pandemic in America has been a perfect storm of bad beginnings. In addition to an unprecedented growth in our population's density and mobility—both in America and around the world—we are a populace wrestling with a variety of environmental and sociological stressors.

What's more, America has been afflicted, especially in the first year of the pandemic, by fundamental elements from each of the worst human pandemics—1) an American president who bore a discomforting resemblance to the Emperor Justinian, 2) a nationalist/evangelical oligarchy that has held America in a reverent thrall similar to the grip in which the medieval Roman Church held Europe, 3) a hodgepodge of ethnicities jockeying for ascendance, much like the nations of pre-Columbian America, and 4) a virtual war between two global adversaries—the U.S. and China—who esteemed competition over compassion until a lethal virus was set loose upon the world.

Many current writers seem addicted to using the word "unprecedented" when they describe the coronavirus pandemic in America. George Santayana would rub all their noses in the historical evidence, exhorting them to recognize that we Americans are *awash* in pandemic precedents. We are just too ignorant or arrogant to remember these precedents and put them to productive use.

True, all pandemics have been made worse by humankind's bull-headed denial and delusions of omnipotence...or at least by our excessive confidence in our ability to prevail over Nature. But the train wreck of coincidence that has led to the coronavirus pandemic is several orders of magnitude beyond what anyone has, or could have, predicted. We *must* learn from the collective pandemic past when navigating our present and planning our future if we wish to avoid repeating those disasters.

And yet, it is important to recognize that this has been a perfect storm of bad beginnings...a tangle of awful circumstances for the human race. The source of that dark synchronicity must remain a mystery for now, and perhaps it will remain so forever...just as we will never know why the three weird sisters had to accost Macbeth at the beginning of his tragic story.

With such mysterious beginnings, we must first *tell* the story. Then, if we are patient and wise, we might be fortunate enough to discern some meaning in the story we have told by the time the curtain comes down.

So let's continue our story by introducing the invader-protagonist of our tale...

CHAPTER 2

Let's Meet Our Most Deadly Pandemic Invaders

The Novel Coronavirus and Its Predecessors

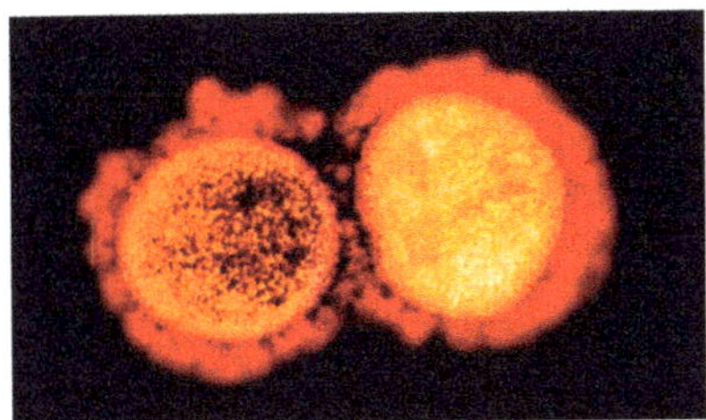

SARS-CoV-2 virus (NIAID)

But what about the courage
of the cancer cell
that breaks out from the crowd
it has belonged to all its life

like a housewife erupting
from her line at the grocery store
because she just can't stand
the sameness anymore?

What about the virus that arrives
in town like a traveler
from somewhere faraway
with suitcases in hand,

who only wants a place
to stay, a chance to get ahead
in the land of opportunity,
but who smells bad,

talks funny, and reproduces fast?
What about the microbe that
hurls its tiny boat straight
into the rushing metabolic tide,

no less cunning and intrepid
than Odysseus; that gambles all
to found a city
on an unknown shore?

What about their bill of rights,
their access to a full-scale,
first-class destiny?
their chance to realize

maximum potential?-which, sure,
will come at the expense
of someone else, someone
who, from a certain point of view,

is a secondary character,
whose weeping is almost
too far off to hear,

a noise among the noises
coming from the shadows
of any brave new world.

– **Tony Hoagland**[12]

12. Hoagland, Tony. "Brave World" from *Donkey Gospel.* Minneapolis, MN: Graywolf Press, 1998. Copyright © 1998 by Tony Hoagland. Reprinted with the permission of The Permissions Company, LLC on behalf of Graywolf Press, Minneapolis, Minnesota, graywolfpress.org.

We want to believe that the most powerful invaders in our deadliest stories of conquest are the ones who have colorful personalities, dramatic style, and compelling motivations. We presume they have clever schemes, wily skills, and dauntless courage.

Not true.

In the history of our world, the deadliest invaders have been the ones whose character profiles were so simple and miniscule that they were literally undetectable. Undetectable, that is, until we were forced to surrender to those murderers the precious field of combat…our bodies. And often, our lives. And sometimes for entire centuries.

I'm talking about the viruses and bacteria that have outnumbered and outgunned us since the dawn of time.

Although microorganisms were not seen by human eyes until the 17th century CE, they were actually among the first life forms on Earth, emerging from the chemical soup of our planet's origins about 3.5 billion years ago. In other words, if the history of Earth were compressed into a year, bacteria and viruses appeared in the equivalent of February. By contrast, we humans appeared on December 31...in the last second before midnight. Guess who has more experience at surviving and thriving?

And the thing that makes it even harder to profile the invader in our current pandemic story is the fact that, like many microorganisms, the novel coronavirus isn't even *alive*. That's right—viruses are technically not living things. They can only be "viable," and then only when they make land on the fertile soil of a compatible host…like the human body. This means that viruses can lie dormant for many years, and then wake up (or "resume viability") when they begin to colonize their biologically-mandated hosts.

As for describing anything like goals or motivation for our infectious invader… Well, it must be admitted that the goals of microorganisms like viruses and bacteria are *extremely* simple, as one might expect for extremely tiny things. Their invasion campaign is much more like a chemical compulsion than a chosen goal. In other words, when a virus or bacillus makes camp in our bodies, *it is **only** doing the **only** thing it **can** do.* It's rather like the way sugar *must* dissolve when it is placed in water. The behavior of a virus or bacillus is essentially chemical karma.

Thus, there is only *one* motivation, *one* option, *one* life plan for a virus or bacillus—to locate a hospitable environment and then replicate for as long as possible. Locate and replicate...replicate...replicate...until the same forces of biology that programmed its compulsive existence somehow compel its termination.

Simplicity like that definitely limits one's career options. But it also prevents *anything* from shifting one's focus. No getting distracted by the urge to go to Starbucks. No worrying about the unpaid rent or the tragic state of one's love life. The absolute focus of a microorganism is infinitely beyond anything a human can muster, and that monomaniacal focus is a decisive advantage in the competition to prevail.

In addition, microorganisms have the advantage of being *extremely* small. On the *point* of a pin, you could pack one million *large* bacteria. And a virus is 1,000 times smaller than a bacillus. That means one *billion* viruses can fit on the *point* of a pin. Those big blobs under the heading of this chapter? One billion of them can dance on the tip of the sharpest pin. It's quite incomprehensible, isn't it?

Well, extremely small things are very difficult for *most* of us to comprehend, let alone fight. We're pretty effective combatants when we encounter opponents that we can see, grab, and punch in the nose. But fighting extremely small things that we can't even *see* is like wrestling with phantoms. Which is probably why the history of medicine often reads like ghostbusting—full of weird contraptions and fantastic notions. Come to think of it, the diseases caused by invisible microorganisms *still* evoke some pretty unscientific responses in a lot of people. These are the people who act as if contagious diseases aren't real, and *really* dangerous, simply because germs can't be clobbered with a brick.

Of course, we've always had *evidence* of our pandemic invaders, because we've been suffering and dying from their effects for millennia. But for most of those millennia, we've been blaming our microbial afflictions on demons, foreigners, and the disadvantaged members of our communities. ("The Devil brought the plague!" "The flu came from the Spaniards!" "The Jews poisoned the wells with cholera!")

Given the hysteria that our invisible invaders ignite, it's rather astonishing that practical countermeasures for epidemic disease were *ever* developed. But in fact, social distancing was implemented as far back as the 6th century CE, and the use of fire was an ancient attempt to drive off the aspiring colonizers of our bodies. We have been attempting to banish or embargo our microscopic invaders for centuries. But we've usually been less successful at defeating our pandemic diseases than they have been at colonizing and laying waste to our bodies.

So when were we actually able to *see* the ambitious adventurers of the sub-visible world? Well, bacteria were first observed in 1676 by Antoni van Leeuwenhoek, using a microscope he made himself. Viruses, on the other hand, were not observed until 1931, upon the invention of the electron microscope by Ernst Ruska. Yes, that's right. The doctors and scientists who fought the 1918 flu epidemic never knew that they were fighting something that was a thousand times smaller than a bacillus, which was the smallest microorganism that they could see.

And it wasn't until 2011 that the nanoscope was invented, which permits us to see active viruses in natural light without the use of dye. Hence, the coronavirus photo under this chapter heading was made possible only twelve years ago. These microscopic critters may be simple to the point of absurdity, but their miniscule size and ancient subtlety makes them formidable invaders in any story that transpires on our gargantuan human scale. A story like, say, a global pandemic.

Of course, viruses and bacteria can *never* be said to possess personality traits, any more than they possess dreams, dreads, or grudges. But they *can* be said to have distinct profiles. Specifically, microorganisms are *not* all the same. They may not have conscious goals, but they *do* have different chemical destinies. They may not have character flaws, but they *do* have unique vulnerabilities. They may not have acquired talents, but they *do* have evolved specialties. And they may not have the capacity to learn new skills, but they *do* have the adaptive advantages that come with lightning-fast replication, billions of years' worth of adaptative evolution, and populations in the centillions—or 1×100^{300}—which is just my extravagant way of expressing what is actually an uncountable number.

In other words, our micro-invaders are playing by rules that most of us can barely understand. And they are highly skilled at tactics that we can only occasionally counteract...and even then, not very well. Viruses and bacteria are hindered by the physical mandates of their functional simplicity, but they are vastly aided by their ancient history, their infinite numbers, and their mandate to pursue their chemical karma until they are contained or eradicated by opposing chemical laws.

We often refer to our microscopic invaders as "bugs," because those are the smallest *visible* things that seem to us most similar to microorganisms in their roles and habits. And there have been recent comparisons of microorganisms to the mythic characters we call "zombies," because of their irresistible mandate to feed upon living humans. But in the end, viruses and bacteria are fundamentally the stuff of our own human history. They are our ancestors and our fellow Earthlings, our beginnings and our ends. They are around us and inside us, as they always have been. And when we die, by their actions or any other, microorganisms are there to receive us and transform us back into earth.

Now that we have a sense of the characters that pandemic pathogens are destined to be, let's meet our current protagonist, the novel coronavirus, and the pathogens who have come before it in pandemic history...

♦ ♦ ♦

Bats. They say it began its epic pilgrimage in bats. And it *may* have made a stopover inside of an animal called a "pangolin"—a creature almost as improbable as the virus itself. Or it may have been delivered by some Frankensteinian midwifery in a Chinese virus lab (sigh).

Wherever it came from, the novel coronavirus isn't *entirely* novel. It has coronavirus cousins...*hundreds* of them. But only seven coronaviruses have discovered humans to be hospitable soil for colonization, and only three of those seven have caused serious problems for the brave worlds of human flesh upon which they have made land. There was the original Severe Acute Respiratory Syndrome (aka SARS-1), which planted its microscopic flag on human soil in 2002 and killed 812 of its hosts. Next came Middle East Respiratory Syndrome (aka MERS), making camp in human flesh in 2012 and killing 866 of its hosts.

And now we have Severe Acute Respiratory Syndrome, Coronavirus 2 (aka SARS-CoV-2), which lightly reared its spherical head in December 2019 and hit the big time a mere three months later. That's when the World Health Organization assigned the exalted status of "global pandemic" to its pathogenic progeny, Covid-19.

The novel coronavirus is still infecting millions, and as of June 2022, it has killed well over five million people...or possibly three times that number.[13] It will eventually kill many more, because its campaign of colonization continues to surge around the world. Yes indeed, our micro-invader has come a long way from its humble debut, either in the wet markets of Wuhan or in the Wuhan Institute of Virology. As the television pundit Trevor Noah has aptly declared, "For corona, this is pretty cool...it's like going platinum!"[14] Mind you, corona's triumph is a millennial catastrophe for those of us who are its "secondary characters," as Tony Hoagland refers to us in the poem that started this chapter. Well, it's all a matter of perspective, isn't it?

13. "Covid results briefing." *Institute for Health Metrics and* Evaluation, May 6, 2021. https://www.healthdata.org/sites/default/files/files/Projects/COVID/2021/95_briefing_United_Kingdom_11.pdf

14. *The Daily Show with Trevor Noah*, Broadcast by Comedy Central on March 11, 2020. https://www.cc.com/episodes/7ktfsd/the-daily-show-with-trevor-noah-extended-march-11-2020-bill-de-blasio-dave-burd-season-25-ep-74

From any perspective, novel coronavirus is a virtuoso. In the terms of Hoagland's poem, this little critter is not only colonizing its brave new world of humanity, it is conquering and transforming it. Microbiologically speaking, you have to admire its pluck and persistence. Too bad about the legions of dispossessed, disabled, and dead humans it is leaving in its wake…

I'm being sardonic, of course, but that's because there are tragedies that can only be conveyed with black humor, especially if we want to avoid being anesthetized by dehumanizing statistics. I am attempting, after all, to profile a mass murderer who is not itself a living thing. To repeat, a virus is only "viable"—not alive—when it is colonizing a host. And as I also said earlier, there is no intent in this serial killer, because there is no intent in *any* pandemic pathogen. It is simply compelled by chemical laws to fulfill its biochemical mandate. Nonetheless, it seems important that we get acquainted with this viral entity, because its mandate is so subtle, agile, and globally cataclysmic.

♦ ♦ ♦

At the risk of remaining sardonic for another paragraph, let me start by comparing the novel coronavirus to its chief contenders for Most Deadly Pandemic Invader in Human History. In terms of sweeping contagion and devastating mortality, those contenders would have to be the three diseases we met in the preceding chapter:

1. Plague (*a.k.a.* the bacillus *yersinia pestis*)
2. Smallpox (*a.k.a.* the virus *variola major*)
3. The 1918 flu (*a.k.a.* the virus *influenzavirus A, type H1N1*)

Let's get to know these micro-invaders and compare them to novel coronavirus.

PLAGUE

Ring around the rosie,
A pocket full of posies.
Ashes, ashes,
We...all...fall...down!

– 14th Century children's song about the plague

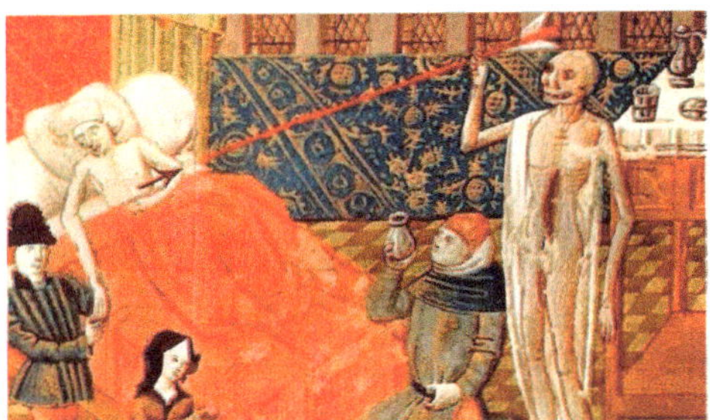

Death of a noble person by plague, 15th century (Wikimedia)

The history of plague as a colonizer of humanity is ancient, but it could be argued that it remains horribly alive in our racial memories. We have called plague by a variety of colorful names, all of which denote the terror that it has inspired in our species since *yersinia pestis* first made camp in a prehistoric human.

"Primal pestilence."

"The Great Mortality."

And of course, "The Black Death."

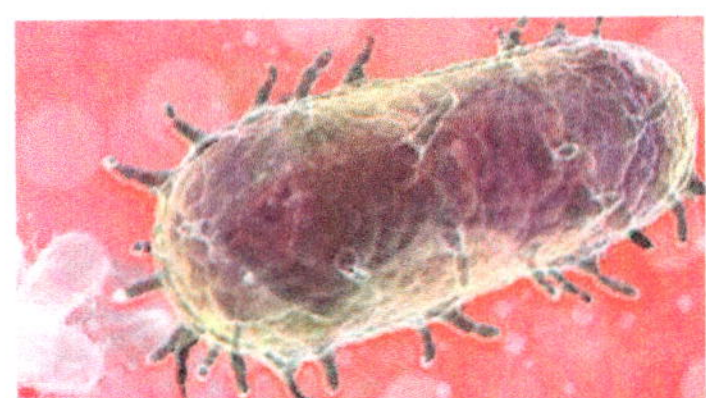

Yersinia pestis (250x Magnification) (CDC)

Plague has found us to be savory hosts as far back as the Late Neolithic and Early Bronze Age, and our world has been ravaged ever since by its epidemic eruptions. The modern form of *yersinia pestis* probably originated about ten thousand years ago, after migrating to the Asia land mass in the bodies of small African rodents. Plague bacteria currently maintain permanent base camps in several natural "reservoirs"—that is, populations of wild ground rodents—where the rodents' high population densities and prolific breeding allow it to thrive without decimating its hosts. The bacillus initially travels from host to host in the gut of the fleas that feed on the rodents, and it comes to feast on humans when our tasty selves come in contact with those plague-infested rodents—rats near all human habitats, but also the marmots of Siberia and the prairie dogs and jackrabbits of North America.

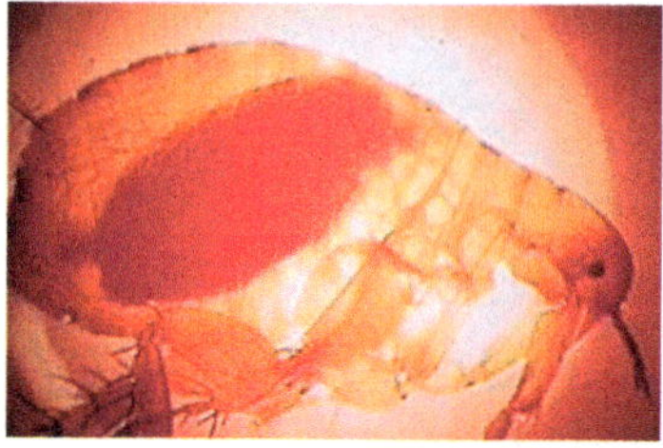

Oriental rat flea (*xenopsylla cheopis)* not yet infected with plague because it is engorged with blood (CDC)

Yersinia pestis had to master some astounding evolutionary gymnastics in order to colonize humans. Especially remarkable is its ability to move among rats via the gut of a flea. It accomplishes this feat by blocking the flea's gut, thereby instigating a ravenous hunger in the infected flea. The starving flea jumps from rat to rat, attempting to draw a meal of blood, but only regurgitating the plague bacteria. The fleas do die off, but not as fast as the rats. And when most of the rats have died of plague, *yersinia pestis* hitches a ride inside the starving fleas as they jump to their next favorite feeding ground... human beings.[15] [16]

The creativity of the plague bacillus is, however, largely confined to its method of contagion. Once inside the human body, plague has only three operating protocols, and these appear to have remained constant throughout the millennia that plague has tormented and annihilated its human victims.

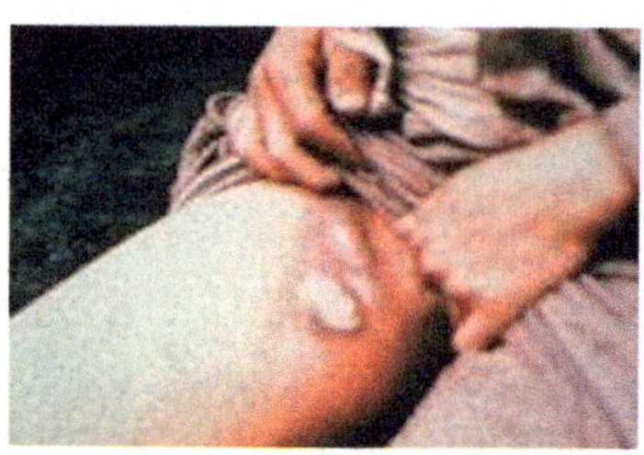

Plague bubo (CDC)

Bubonic plague is the most common manifestation of *yersinia pestis*. It enters the host through the bite of a flea, who regurgitates the bacteria as it attempts (again, in vain) to feed on the blood of the creature it is biting. The bacteria travel with our white cells, which are called into action by our body's immune system, and this allows the plague bacteria to whisk through our lymph system and set up camp in our lymph nodes, primarily under our arms and in our groin.

15. A brilliant and highly readable description of this process, as well as the entire history of *yersinia pestis,* is available in William Rosen's *Justinian's Flea: The First Great Plague and the End of the Roman Empire.* New York: Penguin, 2008, pp 167-198.

16. Piret, Jocelyne and Guy Bolvin. "Pandemics throughout History." *Frontiers in Microbiology*, January 15, 2021. https://www.frontiersin.org/articles/10.3389/fmicb.2020.631736/full

Once ensconced in our lymph nodes, the bacteria burst into action, exploding like a firebomb as they expand the nodes into the "buboes" that give the disease its name. Later, the bacteria travel throughout our vascular system, triggering hemorrhage in the extremities and other parts of our body. These hemorrhagic sites darken to black, and death usually follows soon thereafter. The "black" in Black Death is not just a metaphor. The extremities of plague victims literally turn black before they die.

A terminal victim of ***bubonic plague*** dies in about eight days. However, in cases of ***pneumonic plague,*** where *yersinia pestis* infects the lungs directly (when other plague victims exhale bacteria in their later stages), or in cases of ***septicemic plague,*** where the bacteria enter directly into the bloodstream, a huge majority of the victims die, usually within 24 hours from the time of infection.

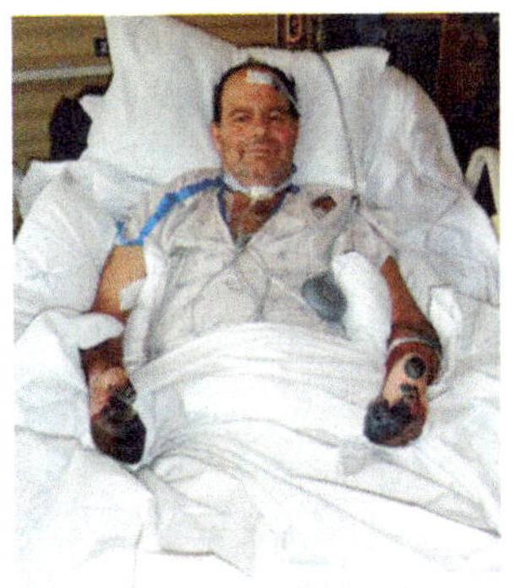

Plague victim in Prineville, Oregon, USA (2012) (AP Photo/The Gaylord Family)

It is estimated that *yersinia pestis* is capable of killing 50% of its adult victims and an even greater percentage of its child victims, especially without the antibiotic treatment that must be administered in early stages of infection. And 10% of its victims die even *with* antibiotic treatment.

Plague is our most ancient pandemic colonizer, and although it has not been able to launch a successful pandemic campaign in human flesh since the beginning of the 20th century, it dwells perpetually in the ground rodent population of central Asia and the central United States...as the American in the photo learned when he tried to remove a plague-infected mouse from the mouth of his cat. (Yes, he survived, but his fingers and toes had to be amputated.)

Bacteria have no conscious manifesto, but their biological mandate is as simple and explicit as their biological structure. And in the millennia before the invention of the microscope, it was also a great advantage to be very, very small in comparison to the host that one was destined to colonize. It's hard to be targeted or deterred, much less eradicated, when you're invisible.

SMALLPOX

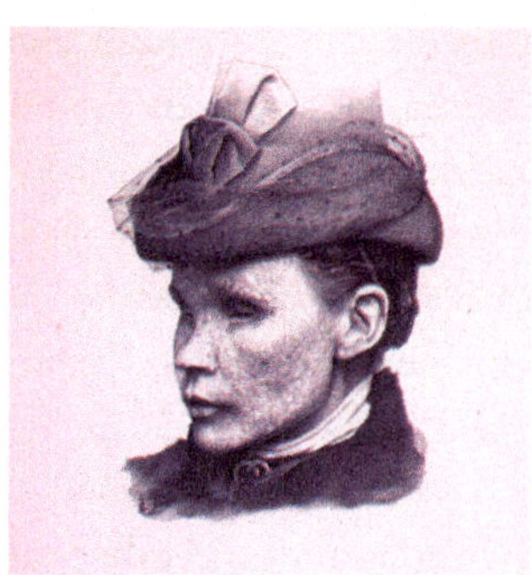

Survivor of Smallpox (National Library of Medicine)

See the malign envenom'd Pain
Shoot thro' ev'ry tainted Vein!
With hostile Force the Flames engage,
And feed the growing Fever's Rage:
Thro' ev'ry Artery they burn,
And to consume that Heart conspire
That glow'd with a more gen'rous Fire.

– Henry Travers
Upon Cœlia Sick of the Small Pox[17]

Small as *yersinia pestis* is, the plague bacillus is *gigantic* when compared to its prime historical competitor for Most Deadly Pandemic Invader...*variola major,* also known as "smallpox." Called by a variety of horrible epithets—"the burning scourge," "the speckled monster," and most ominously, "the Devil's pox"—smallpox was the dread and constant companion of humanity for millennia.

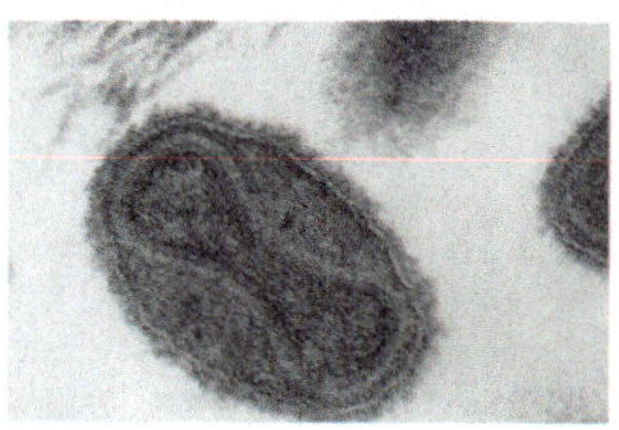

Smallpox virus (370KxMagnification) (CDC)

Although there is debate about the first human case of smallpox (600 BCE? 1500 BCE?), most scientists believe that smallpox afflicted humans long before the birth of Christ. Most scientists further believe that smallpox came to us through an African rodent about 10,000 years ago, much like plague. And most scientists would *like* to believe that smallpox has been eradicated from the Earth, officially as of 1980.

But most scientists also realize that viruses are *not* living things, as bacteria are. As we've already learned, viruses are capable of lying dormant, and potentially viable, for a *very* long time, even in conditions that would kill living things like bacteria. So let's not get too smug about the eradication of smallpox. Few things in nature go gentle into that good night of oblivion...especially the really *little* things.

In terms of sheer scariness, you'd be hard pressed to find a more terrifying

17. Travers, Henry. *Miscellaneous Poems and Translations.* London: Benjamin Motte, 1731, #56. https://xtf.lib.virginia.edu/xtf/view?docId=chadwyck_ep/uvaGenText/tei/chep_2.0879.xml;chunk.id=d12;toc.depth=1;toc.id=d3;brand=default

invader than smallpox for an epidemic story. (Well, except maybe plague, but who wants to quibble about comparative horrors?) Agonizing, disfiguring, highly contagious, and blazingly lethal, *smallpox killed 300 million people in just the first 75 years of the 20th century.* We have no idea how many people have died from smallpox, but we do know that among the humans it has colonized, it has killed approximately 40% of its adult hosts and 80% of its child hosts within a month, and often within two weeks from their symptoms' onset.

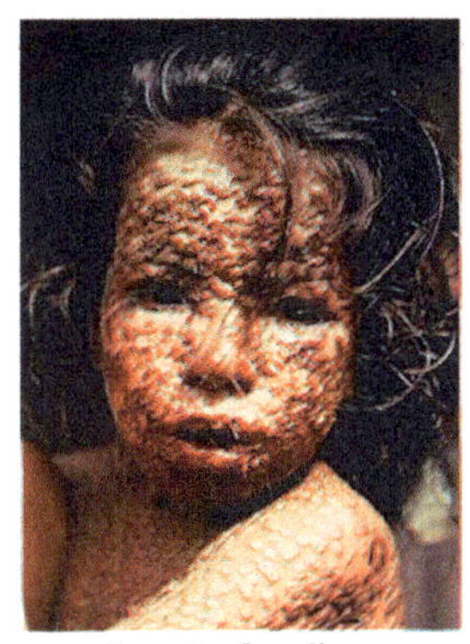

Portrait of smallpox in a child (CDC)

In terms of its modes of transmission, smallpox is a wizard of infection, travelling on any droplet, scab, mucous, exhalation, or effluvia from an infected person. But once it has made land in a human body, smallpox is something of a dullard, especially as compared to novel coronavirus. Smallpox can hitch a ride on a variety of transports from one host to another, and it can make land on a variety of locations in its new host. But after it begins to colonize a human, it always proceeds the same way.

For about three days, smallpox starts out like the flu, including fever, malaise, and digestive symptoms. Within a few more days, the person's temperature drops to normal and the first lesions appear on mucous membranes of the mouth, tongue, and throat. These lesions quickly grow and rupture, releasing large amounts of virus into the saliva. Promptly, the fearsome skin lesions appear on the person's face, spreading to the whole body within 48 hours and either killing or maiming the victim within the next two weeks. Those who died were in agony, while those who survived were left horribly disfigured and often blind.

This is a pandemic invader that has ignited mass terror, inflicted hideous suffering, and decimated entire populations. Its only weakness was that it could annihilate its brave new worlds as quickly as it colonized them, destroying the hosts upon which it depended. Smallpox could incinerate an entire society, but it could also flame out. Afterward, it would depend on travelers to carry its glowing embers of latent virus to new lands of "virgin" flesh for another conquest. Sadly, smallpox regularly found forests of humanity that could fuel its firestorms for generations...as we have learned from the devastating story of the post-Columbian pandemics in the New World.

THE 1918 FLU

I had a little bird and her name was Enza.
I opened up the window, and in-flu-enza.

– Children's jump rope rhyme in 1918
(Children under five had the second highest mortality rate from the 1918 flu, after the elderly)

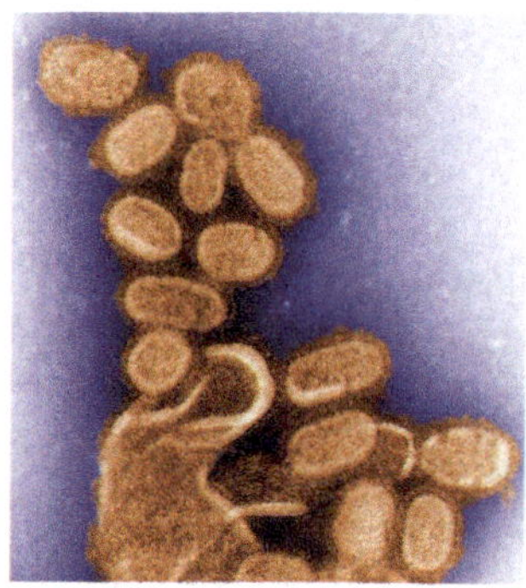

Reconstructed 1918 H1N1 virus 370KxMagnification (CDC)

Scientists believe that the family of viruses that contains *influenzavirus A* probably migrated from birds to humans around 10,000 years ago. Specifically, the flu viruses have been with us ever since we domesticated fowl for breeding and consumption. Like the smallpox virus, these influenza critters are incomprehensibly small—a thousand times smaller than bacteria—and most of them are non-lethal nuisances. But in the years leading up to 1918, one of those infinitesimal critters made the leap from birds (a Kansas chicken, probably) to pigs (again, in Kansas). And in 1918, the virus made its final jump from porcine to human soil, and the rest is pandemic history.

Influenza viruses are pretty malleable when it comes to mutating and evolving. Some very recent research indicates that the initial form of *influenzavirus A, Type H1N1*—the one that traveled with the doughboys in March 1918 to WWI—was not exactly the same as the H1N1 that returned to America a few months later.[18] This is consistent with the fact that after a relatively unremarkable start in the spring of 1918, H1N1 began a spree of human destruction that began in August 1918 and eclipsed all prior pandemics for speed of lethality. In the space of eighteen months, H1N1 spread to every corner of the globe, *infecting at least 50% of all humanity*, and precipitating the deaths of between 50 and 100 million of its hosts. Some of its victims died of secondary pneumonia, which was lethal in the days before antibiotics. But H1N1 itself was deadly in a way that had never before been seen in a virus. In the end, 675,000 Americans died of the 1918

18. Zhang, Sarah "A clue to why the 1918 pandemic came back stronger than before." *The Atlantic*, May 24, 2021. https://www.theatlantic.com/science/archive/2021/05/pandemic-virus-mutations-1918-flu/618972/

flu, and far more soldiers *on all sides of the war* died of the flu than were killed by combat. It has been persuasively argued that H1N1 ended World War I long before it would otherwise have concluded.

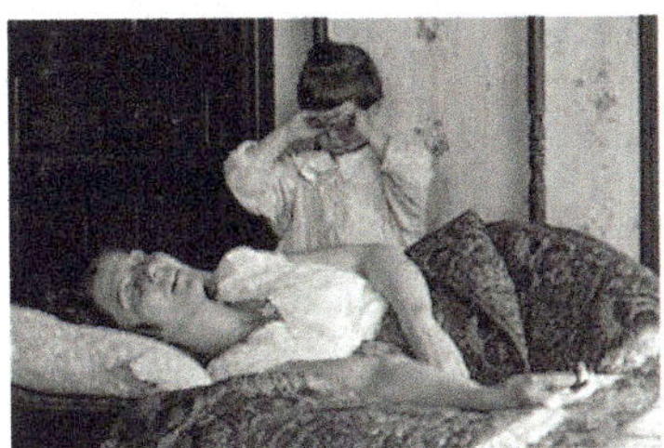

Child sobbing for her mortally ill sister in 1918 (Library of Congress)

H1N1 was not as creative as novel coronavirus, attacking the respiratory system as all flus do. But the novel thing that it *did* do for its time was to kill young, strong adults, as well as the babies and elderly people that influenzas normally kill. It is estimated that H1N1 killed 25 million of its human hosts within its first 25 *weeks*. (By contrast, HIV/AIDS killed 25 million people in its first 25 *years*.) Although it is true that all deaths are mourned equally, such vast mortality in such a short time is nearly inconceivable. But more on that later, when we discuss the effects that these pathogenic invaders had on their victims' bodies and their survivors' psyches.

For the moment, we can only be thankful that influenzas are relatively vulnerable to seasonal conditions, preferring the winter months for most parts of the world. And even more fortunate is the fact that H1N1 appears to have mutated from its 1918 form into something slightly less catastrophic by the time it flamed out in 1920. However, Nature thrives on the dance between stability and change, so mutations are happening every day. And mutations that have been done can conceivably be *un*done. Certainly, during the hundred years when we have mostly forgotten about H1N1, H1N1 has *not* forgotten about *us*. It has not yet managed to achieve its original lethality, *but every flu pandemic since 1918 has been inflicted by a descendent of the 1918 H1N1 virus*.[19]

NOVEL CORONAVIRUS

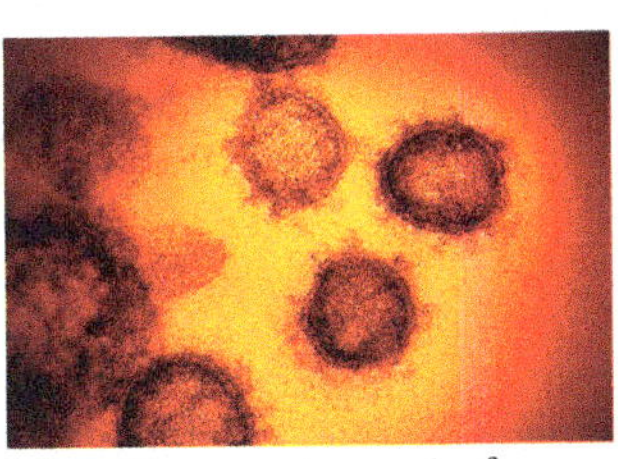

Electron micrograph of SARS-CoV2 virus (NIAID)

Each man's death diminishes me,
For I am involved in mankind.
Therefore, send not to know
For whom the bell tolls.
It tolls for thee.

– **John Donne, *Meditation XVII,* 1624**

19. Morens, David M., Jeffery K. Taubenberger, and Anthony S. Fauci. "The persistent legacy of the 1918 influenza virus." *The New England Journal of Medicine,* July 16, 2009, pp 225-229. https://www.nejm.org/doi/full/10.1056/nejmp0904819

They named it SARS-CoV-2—Severe Respiratory Virus, Coronavirus 2—because the respiratory system was its first noticeable port of entry in most of its initial human hosts. But later, scientists and physicians noticed that its victims were getting sick (and sometimes not so sick) in a variety of ways that weren't respiratory at all. Kidney failure, liver failure, gastrointestinal disorders, multiple brain dysfunctions, diverse cardiac problems, and uncontrollable strokes as a result of blood clots large and small, plus a systemic inflammatory syndrome in children that had only rarely been seen before.

In the end, the viral investigators concluded that novel coronavirus is fundamentally a *vascular* disease.[20] Yes, it normally arrives through our respiratory systems. But it quickly battens upon vascular cells and uses our circulatory system as a means of high-speed transport, leapfrogging around the entire body as it locks onto the ACE2 receptors (officially *angiotensin-converting enzymes*-2) that line all of our blood vessels and proliferate in most of our vital organs.

True, the novel coronavirus initially makes its most noticeable mischief in our respiratory systems, sometimes causing dangerously low blood oxygen levels without even letting our bodies notice what's happening. But because those little ACE2 receptors are located just about everywhere that matters inside of us, and because the spike on the coronavirus acts like a key to unlock the ACE2 receptors, it's like giving this pandemic invader a passkey to go nearly anywhere it wants in the human body. Nothing stops it...unless it happens to encounter just the right mix of opposing immune responses, which it usually does *not*.[21] Imagine giving the master key of your house to a home invader. Anything can happen and probably will...and none of it good.

Once the coronavirus has unlocked and entered an ACE2 enzyme, it can replicate at an astonishing rate, until the enzyme erupts with a host of coronavirus replicants, all of whom are armed with the same master keys to the kingdom. And off they go!

Now that we are well into the pandemic, we have learned that SARS-CoV-2 is able to reside—quietly at first, but disastrously later on—in our kidneys, liver, intestines, nervous systems, and hearts, as well in our lungs. And the

20. Smith, Dana G. "Covid-19 may be a blood vessel disease, which explains everything." *Elemental*, May 28, 2020. https://elemental.medium.com/coronavirus-may-be-a-blood-vessel-disease-which-explains-everything-2c4032481ab2

21. Srinam, Krishna, Paul Insel, and Rohit Loomba. "What is the ACE2 receptor, how is it connected to coronavirus, and why might it be key to treating COVID-19? The experts explain." *The Conversation*, May 14, 2020. https://theconversation.com/what-is-the-ace2-receptor-how-is-it-connected-to-coronavirus-and-why-might-it-be-key-to-treating-covid-19-the-experts-explain-13692

chaos it can create in our vascular network and immune system can wreak several kinds of secondary havoc in our brains. Sometimes the virus sets up a base camp (or even buys a condo) in just one organ. But sometimes it moves from organ to organ, like a viral Goldilocks seeking the "just right" place for its new home, while leaving rubble and wreckage in its wake.

Yes indeed, SARS-CoV-2 is a nimble critter, as variable and unpredictable as it is tenacious. As it camps and decamps around the body, the virus leaves a trail of symptoms that are, at the least, bewildering and frightening. But in many cases, those symptoms are permanently debilitating, and in the worst cases, lethally devastating. We will talk more about why all these symptoms arise when we discuss the defenders of our human soil, but the short version is that along with possessing the master key to gain access to our entire circulatory systems and most of our crucial organs, the novel coronavirus can trigger a collision of immune responses that produce a maelstrom of bleeding and clotting. This biochemical chaos is tragically ineffective when it comes to evicting the viral colonizer. Even more tragically, this immune response itself can quickly lead to the death of the body it is protecting.

At this point, it seems that novel coronavirus is killing about 4% of its human hosts worldwide—which is more than double the kill rate for the 1918 flu. But because this virus kills more slowly than H1N1 flu, we will not know the sum of its destruction for years to come. And we are even farther from knowing the full extent of long-term damage the virus leaves behind in those who have survived its colonization attempts. However, in the time since it first made land on human terrain, we have learned that the virus appears to cause lasting physical and cognitive impairments in one out of eight patients, in a syndrome referred to as "long Covid."[22] [23] For example, *the chest x-rays of asymptomatic Covid survivors look worse than the x-rays of heavy smokers.*[24] Doctors are also reporting inexplicably high rates of diabetes onset in otherwise healthy people who have technically recovered from Covid.[25] More disturbing is the high rate of cardiac and

22. Raveendran, A.V., Rajeev Jayadevan, and S. Sashidharan. "Long Covid: An Overview." *Diabetes and Metabolic Syndrome: Research and Reviews.* May-June 2021, pp 869-875. https://www.sciencedirect.com/science/article/pii/S1871402121001193?via%3Dihub

23. Ballering, Aranka, Sander van Zon, Tim Hartman, and Judith Rosmalen. "Persistence of somatic symptoms after COVID-19 in the Netherlands: an observational cohort study." *Lancet*, August 6, 2022, Vol. 400, Issue 10350. https://doi.org/10.1016/S0140-6736(22)01214-4

24. Gowdy, ShaCamree. "Texas trauma doctor says post-Covid lungs are more damaged than smokers." *Houston Chronicle*, January 15, 2021. https://www.sfchronicle.com/coronavirus/article/Post-Covid19-lungs-smokers-Texas-15873888.php

25. Blakemore, Erin. "New diabetes cases linked to covid-19". *Washington Post*, February 1, 2021. https://www.washingtonpost.com/health/2021/02/01/covid-new-onset-diabetes/

brain dysfunction in post-Covid patients, even those whose Covid infections seemed mild, and even months after the infections appeared to clear.[26] [27] And perhaps most disturbing of all is the recent finding that people over 65 who have had Covid (and recovered) are significantly more likely to develop Alzheimer's disease.[28]

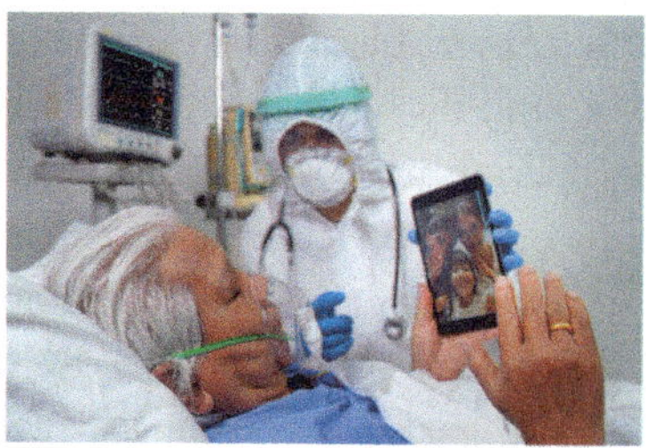

Covid patients are given phones and iPads to communicate with family members, often for the last time. (Shutterstock, model-signed release)

Among the three coronaviruses that have been able to colonize humans, there is no doubt that SARS Cov-2 is the prodigy of its clan. And it's likely to have a meteoric run in its campaign of colonization because it displays *all* of the most successful components of pandemic diseases. Indeed, *novel coronavirus displays more successful components, combined in a single pandemic invader, than any disease that humanity has ever encountered*:

1. It is highly contagious.
2. It is not highly lethal, so it doesn't burn up its hosts before it can be transmitted.
3. It can take a long time to stimulate the host's immune system into manifesting symptoms, so the host is often contagious long before they know it. In fact, novel coronavirus doesn't provoke *any* noticeable symptoms in some hosts, so the host is contagious without ever realizing they have been infected.
4. Unlike every other human disease of pandemic proportions, once novel coronavirus makes land inside a human body, it is astonishingly variable in its replication sites.
5. It remains unclear when, exactly, we start and stop being contagious.

26. Cha, Ariana E. "Experts projecting a 'tidal wave' of cardiovascular cases related directly and indirectly to the coronavirus." *Washington Post*, February 21, 2022. https://www.washingtonpost.com/health/2022/02/21/covid-cardiac-issues-longterm/

27. Ely, Wes. "How long Covid reshapes the brain—and how we might treat it." *Washington Post*, August 25, 2022. https://www.washingtonpost.com/outlook/2022/08/25/long-covid-brain-science-fog-recovery/

28. Wang, Lindsey, Pamela Davis, Nora Volkow, Nathan Berger, David Kaelber, and Rong Xu. "Association of COVID-19 with new-onset Alzheimer's disease." *Journal of Alzheimer's Disease*, 89 (2022), 411-414.

6. If a person manages to survive Covid, it is clear that survival no longer confers immunity. There are now many cases in which Covid survivors have been re-infected by the virus, especially since the advent of the Omicron variant.
7. Finally, although this coronavirus is not as mutable as an influenza virus, it still has vast mutation capacity because it is infecting a large portion of the 7.8 billion humans on earth. The deadliest mutations will likely disappear because they will kill off their hosts too quickly (although this didn't stop *influenza H1N1* from killing upwards of 50 million people). But the highly *contagious* mutations will further the success of the virus' colonization, so they are likely to prevail. This is how new strains of novel coronavirus, especially the Delta and Omicron strains, have spread more rapidly around the world.[29]

If a playwright wanted to create a lethal protagonist who was adaptive, resilient, subtle, and disarmingly unpredictable to its victims, it would be hard to craft a more successful invader than novel coronavirus. Despite its infinitesimal size and its lack of qualifications for even being alive, this virus has shown an absolute genius for 1) racing through the world's population, 2) gallivanting around the human body, 3) setting up camp in a variety of body locations, 4) wreaking havoc and sometimes war among the battalions of the body's innate immune responses, and 5) leaving a trail of dead bodies, traumatized people, and surviving hosts who may be candidates for future viral colonization, should the need arise.

Every monumental drama needs a monumental villain, and for all its miniscule stature, novel coronavirus seems perfectly cast for the role of precipitating a global pandemic with profound and enduring consequences. And that being said, every monumental drama also needs more than a setting and an instigator. It needs a heroic *defender*...and usually more than one. These are the characters with whom the invader must do deadly battle in order to prevail. Some defenders are extremely adept at defeating invaders, but other defenders actually end up serving the invader's mission, despite their best intentions and efforts. This dramatic story will be exactly the same.

It is now time for us to meet the defenders who have opposed the novel coronavirus and its pandemic predecessors. Some of these defenders have been highly successful in protecting us against the invaders, while others

29. Molteni, Megan. "Worrisome new coronavirus strains are emerging. Why now?" *Science*, January 27, 2021.

have tragically aided their deadly foes, even as they have earnestly endeavored to defeat them. Yes, the stories of very small and simple entities can be surprisingly complicated and dramatic, producing cataclysmic consequences for their large human hosts.

Let's get to it...

CHAPTER 3

Now Let's Meet Our Fiercest Defenders Against Pandemic Disease

The Body's Immune System, Fighting Fire with Fire

The withering gods of fever swoop down upon us…
– Sophocles, *Oedipus Rex*

Do not curse fever.
In truth, it removes the sins of the children of Adam,
just as a furnace removes dirt from iron.
– Ṣaḥiḥ Muslim, *The Book of Virtues*, #2575

Fever is a mighty engine which nature brings into
the world to the conquest of her enemies.
– Thomas Sydenham, English physician of the 17th century[30]

Every human culture has worshipped a god of fire. And all of our fire gods, since time immemorial, have dealt out life and death in equal measure. Most of our ancient fire gods were volcanic—Hephaestus in Greece, Vulcan in Rome, Hui Li in China, and Agni in Hindu cultures. But even the lightning gods Zeus and Thor were fire gods to their Greek and Norse worshippers. More recently, we've met the Hawai'ian volcano goddess Pele, revered for her capacity to create and destroy the Earth itself. Our fire gods have symbolized the combustible powers of Mother Nature, the ancient deity who could set the world on fire long before we humans could strike the smallest spark. We feared the infernos that Nature created with her lightning, wildfires, and volcanoes, trembling at her destructive heat many millennia before we dared to tame fire for our own purposes.

30. Sydenham, Thomas, and Robert Gordon Latham. *The Works of Thomas Sydenham, MD.* Printed for the Sydenham Society, 1850.

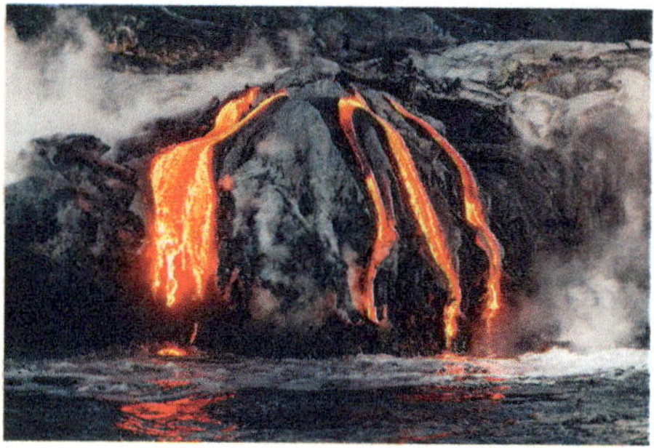

Hawai'ian volcano Kilauea erupting into the Pacific Ocean (Shutterstock)

Similarly, we have regarded with awe the fires that have burned *inside* our human bodies. We are warm-blooded creatures, so we have always known that when our bodies are no longer warm, that means we are no longer alive. And we have also known that when our bodies are excessively hot, we are in some kind of trouble, perhaps deadly trouble. It has always been clear to us that the fires burning inside of us are just as crucial to our survival as the fires that burn outside of us...and sometimes just as dangerous.

Although we have made sweeping advances in our ability to work with many forms of fire, we have never fully mastered its incendiary power—neither outside of our bodies, nor inside of them. Nuclear fires have run amok in our outer world, as have the inner fires of our rages, ambitions, and obsessions. More literally, the inflammatory fires ignited by our immune systems have annihilated us by the millions, with a scope and speed that no external weapon has ever matched. The world is currently facing a biological firestorm that could consume an impressive portion of our species—Covid-19, the progeny of the novel coronavirus. The coronavirus has ignited a host of incendiary consequences, some more metaphorical than fever and inflammation, but no less destructive. The conflagrations of economic catastrophe and emotional despair can burn down civilizations just as effectively as raging fevers and flaming corpses.

But returning to the literal fires of the body, let's consider the fact that all of our pandemic diseases have entailed an element of fire. Fever, abscess, rash, pustule, bubo, and hemorrhage are the fiery agonies that our bodies produce in their effort to defeat a microscopic invader. This is because biological fire is the best weapon the body possesses to fight back against any disease—sometimes to the body's salvation, and sometimes to its miserable demise.

For the ancient Greeks and pre-Roman Etruscans, the god who was responsible for the fires of the body appears to have been Februus, a primal god of purification whose name we memorialize in the month of February. Centuries later, Februus was replaced in Roman culture by a fever goddess called Febris. Febris was both feared and revered, possibly because the ancient Romans witnessed the dual potentials of fever—as a means of killing its human host, but also as a means of killing the disease. Unlike Her predecessor Februus, who was universally malevolent, the female Febris could be benevolent if She chose, so the Romans offered Her gifts and prayers in the hope of bringing forth Her positive powers. Similarly, we now understand that it is often advantageous to allow a fever to run its course, as an effective means of killing off the invading disease.

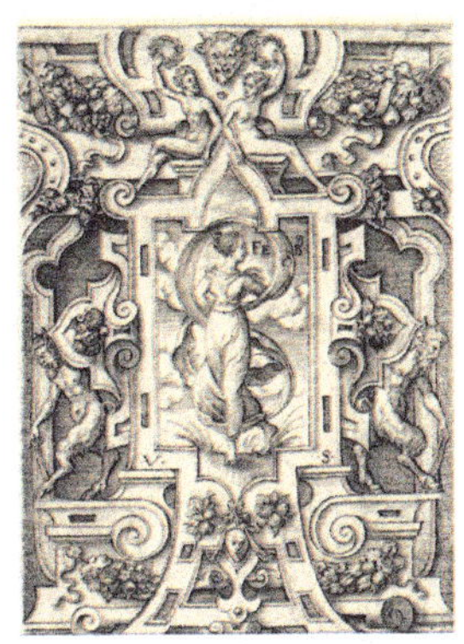

Febris, Virgil Solis (1874) https://www.britishmuseum.org/collection/object/P_1874-0711-1881 (Wikimedia)

For the most part, our ancestors considered the fires of the body to be integral elements of the disease itself, and not (as we now understand them) a part of the body's effort to fight off its microscopic invaders. For the ancients, the fever *was* the disease, so they begged for mercy from fire deities like Febris because they considered them responsible for both the disease and its healing. But in some cultures, sick people have also called upon cooling gods and goddesses to quell the "fires" that were devastating their infected bodies. Let's look at two of these healing "cool ones," as they are called.

In India, the goddess Shitala (शीतला) was, and still is, the deity with the power to cure the diseases of heat—primarily smallpox and other eruptive "heat afflictions." Shitala is usually depicted as riding a white donkey and possessing four arms that enable her to carry her healing implements: 1) a broom for sweeping clean the sickroom, 2) a fan for moving and cooling the dank, overheated air around the patient, 3) a cup of cool water to drink, and 4) a bowl of cool water to cleanse and cool the patient. Shrines to Shitala are still active in India, and her powers are still revered by the Indian people.

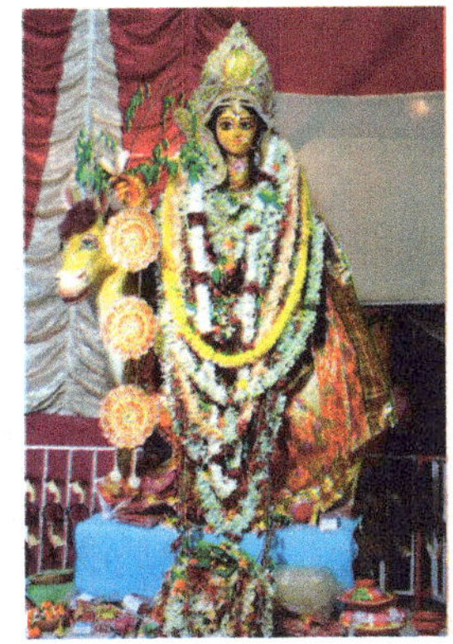

Shitala (शीतला) (Wikimedia)

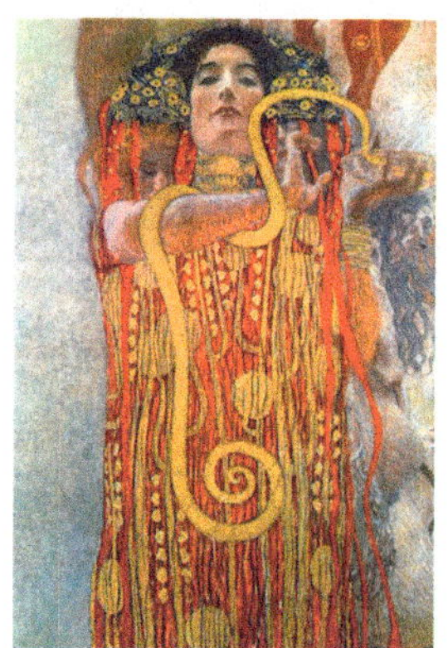
"Hygeia" from *Medicine,* Gustav Klimt (1901) (Wikimedia)

The ancient Greeks revered a similar goddess who carried a bowl of cool water as her means of imbuing good health. This goddess also carried a serpent, an ancient symbol of life force. Her name was Hygeia (Υγεία) and she was the Greek goddess of good health and vitality. For us, Hygeia could be something like the goddess of "good chi" because she healed by enhancing the body's own recuperative powers. She was also invoked to apply her cooling influence to excessive heat, both in the body and in the mind. In other words, Hygeia created good health, psychologically as well as physically, by promoting a calm mind in a cool body. (We assume this is why a temple to Hygeia was located outside of the theater of every great healing center in ancient Greece, recalling the notion that potent stories offer us gifts of healing.[31])

Although many people throughout history have made no distinction between the diseases that have tormented us and the fevers that our bodies ignite to fight those diseases, a few healers have understood that the fires of the body—fever in particular and inflammation in general—are the body's fastest and most effective defenders against any afflictions it has not met before. Admittedly, these fast and fiery weapons are blunt instruments, designed only to be a first line of defense against new invaders. As such, they can sometimes overreact and lead to the death of the body they are defending. But without these ferocious first responders, the body would be a defenseless shore against a host of fiercely determined micro-invaders.

The historical healers who witnessed the body's internal fires often concluded that fire could have the same healing effect when applied externally as internally. For example, the medieval physician Guy de Chauliac may have accomplished the most successful intervention during the Black Death when he instructed Pope Clement VI to isolate himself from everyone and keep fires burning around himself at all times. De Chauliac's understanding about the curative power of fire may not have been scientific by our standards, but Pope Clement's isolation protected him from the pneumonic and septicemic plagues, and the fires that burned continually around him repelled the rats and fleas that transmitted the bubonic form of plague.

31. Pausanias, *Description of Greece (circa 200 A.D.).* Translated by W. H. S. Jones. Cambridge, MA: Harvard University Press, 1973.

Pope Clement survived the Black Death, dying of kidney disease at the relatively advanced age of 62. And in a rare kindness of Fate, de Chauliac himself died of non-plague causes at the exalted age of 68, after preserving the lives of three popes, over two decades, during the worst of the Black Death pandemic.

It would be more than 600 years after de Chauliac's interventions before medical science would identify some of the means by which the human body ignites its own healing "fires"—fires that the body raises in its defense when invaded by aspiring micro-invaders. Sadly, the dangers of using biological fire to wage war *inside* the body are fearfully similar to the dangers of using literal fire as a weapon *outside* of the body. And although the body possesses its own immunological means of cooling, even these cooling countermeasures can have unfortunate, even deadly, consequences.

Despite the potential for fire to burn out of control—inside our bodies as well as outside of them—the firepower that dwells inside us is our most crucial defender. So, let's examine the fires banked within our bodies, awaiting biochemical ignition. These are the fires that can save our bodies... or incinerate them. They are deployed by the microscopic defenders who have assaulted, most immediately and ferociously, every pandemic invader we have ever encountered, fighting as if the existence of their world has depended upon defeating the disease. And usually, it has.

This is the first battalion of defenders who will oppose the deadly invaders in our pandemic dramas—the fierce defenders who comprise our immune systems.

MEETING THE IMMUNE SYSTEM

Be advised;
Heat not a furnace for your foe so hot
That it do singe yourself: we may outrun,
By violent swiftness, that which we run at,
And lose by over-running.

– William Shakespeare and John Fletcher, *Henry VIII*, **I.i**

It is laughable to think that anyone could describe the human immune system in a way that is clear, accurate...and brief. I'm going to try anyway. We simply cannot ignore the most important defenders in every one of our pandemic dramas. And this is especially true in the story of the novel coronavirus, which has had such a confounding influence on the determined warriors of our bi-phasic immune system.

You have already seen the kind of catastrophic damage that can be inflicted by a single viral pathogen like smallpox. Specifically, it has wrought *globally lethal* damage, despite the fact that a virus like smallpox is not even alive, and it is so small that it can join one billion of its kin on the point of a pin. Now imagine a second army of microscopic *defenders*, most of whom are as small and as simple as that single pathogen. This army of infinitesimal defenders is organized into a host of precisely coordinated teams whose only purpose is to detect and destroy the legions of equally infinitesimal invaders that try to make land in our bodies. What's more, each of our microscopic defenders possesses the same singular focus that is held by the microscopic invaders we met in the previous chapter.

This would be like marshalling a synchronized battalion of zombie defenders who are hell-bent on rebuffing daily assaults by battalions of zombie invaders. The defending zombies are determined to annihilate the invaders as much as the invading zombies are determined to colonize the defenders' land. Under these conditions, it is inevitable that raging zombie holocausts would ensue. And in a certain sense, that is exactly what happens during the conflicts between infection and immunity in the human body—thermonuclear zombie war. Just on a microscopic scale.

Welcome to the next chapter of our story—the wars waged by the microscopic defenders who defend us against the pandemic invaders who assault us. The sole focus and purpose of these vigilant defenders is to wage deadly war against all outsiders, including the diseases we met in the prior chapter. Allow me to introduce you to the human immune system, both as it normally functions and as it behaves when it is pitted against four of its deadliest enemies.

The Innate Immune System

There are two major battalions in the immune systems of any animal possessing jaws. (Yes, jaws. That's where the line is drawn. Don't ask me why.) The first battalion is the *innate immune system*, whose mission is to instantly recognize any alien invader and ferociously attack it with the broad-spectrum weapons at its disposal. Specifically, when an enterprising disease makes land on the terrain of our bodies, the first thing that happens (in the best of cases) is that the invader's presence is detected by a host of proteins called *pattern recognition receptors.* These little proteins are like the reconnaissance scouts of our innate immune system, and their job is to determine whether any entity in the body is "self" or "not-self."[32]

When a new arrival is identified as "not-self," these pattern recognition receptors trigger the release of another legion of proteins call *cytokines*. Cytokines mediate between *lots* of body systems, but in the presence of foreign invaders, cytokines function as alarm-activating messengers—rather like microscopic Paul Reveres who broadcast a red alert that alien invaders have landed. In this role, the cytokines communicate between the nervous system and the brain to ignite and regulate the weapons of the innate immune system. (And please remember these little cytokine messenger proteins because they're going to become very important later on. Trust me on this.)

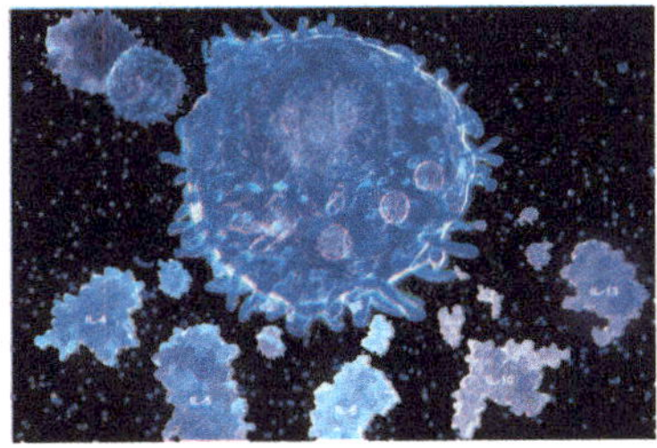

Cytokine protein (Shutterstock)

When the invading disease is mild or moderate, the cytokines send out messages to initiate mild or moderate immune responses. But when the disease is extreme, as in the case of smallpox, the cytokines are activated into what immunologists call a "cytokine storm." The cytokine storm ignites a cascade of dramatic effects that are designed to kick our innate immune defenses into hyperdrive, with the goal of defeating the dangerous disease that is triggering them.

Now, as I mentioned before, the weapons of the innate immune system are pretty blunt instruments, mostly on the order of devouring chemicals (like interferon), biological floods that deluge us with red and white blood cells, and the various fires of inflammation, usually in the form of fever and inflamed tissue. It would be reasonable to compare these front-line immune defenders to the frenzied *berserkers* of Viking legend. The berserkers were the rage-crazed warriors whose killing tactics were modeled after the bear and the wolverine. In other words, the

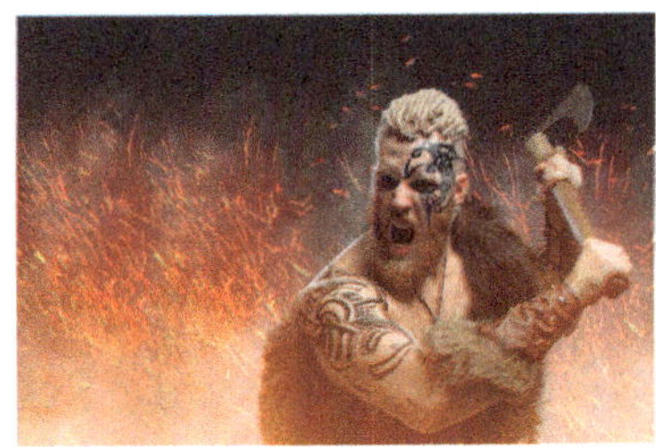

Viking berserker (Shutterstock)

32. And yes, as you might guess, these little pattern recognition receptors can get overzealous, in which case they start telling the immune system that our own body parts are "not-self." Overzealous pattern recognition receptors are usually the inciters of what we call "auto-immune" disorders. So now you know.

warriors of the innate immune system are more like savage firebrands, and very much *not* like a calmly focused sniper. However, what these fiery defenders lack in the sniper's cold calculation and precise aim, they make up for in lightning speed and devastating heat. And their heat is not just metaphorical. Their tactics of fever and inflammation, which we met earlier, are among the most effective weapons in the innate immune system's arsenal.

In other words, these first immune responders are bold and unrefined, microbiologically speaking. But their crucial advantage is that they are *ferocious* and they are *fast*. And when it comes to fighting a new arrival that is invading in one's physical realm, a fierce and speedy response is often the most successful response. It's just like when you're fighting a wildfire. An aggressively rapid response to a small wildfire—even if the response is imprecise and overblown—is much more effective than a precise response initiated long after that small initial fire has erupted into a raging inferno. And this is especially true when you are trying to fight fire *with* fire—in a forest or in a body.

In most cases, the primary battalions of innate immune response serve their purpose of defending our bodies. If they didn't, we would get sick far more often and far more seriously than we do. Consider what happens to people whose innate immune systems have been destroyed or compromised by a debilitating illness or a radical treatment like a bone marrow transplant. A case of the sniffles can kill them.

Even when the fiery tactics of the innate immune system are not sufficient to vanquish the invading disease, they can at least buy our bodies and minds enough time to rally other means of support, both internally and externally. Imprecise and "impulsive" as they may be, the ferocious defenders in our innate immune systems are the reason we can stay alive past infancy.

The Adaptive Immune System

Among our additional sources of *internal* support in the war against disease are the body's second line of immune defense…the *adaptive immune system*. This the legion of warriors that includes the B cell and T cell defenders that some of us remember from the HIV/AIDS epidemic, when this portion of the human immune system was so horribly compromised by the HIV invader.

The "memory" B cells and the "killer" T cells of the adaptive immune system function like a programmed hit squad. They are the specialized assassins who are, on the one hand, the B cells—trained to hold a "memory" of a previously encountered disease—and on the other hand, the "killer" T cells—trained to release the *specific* antibody weapons (proteins) that will destroy the *specific* disease that is their acquired target.

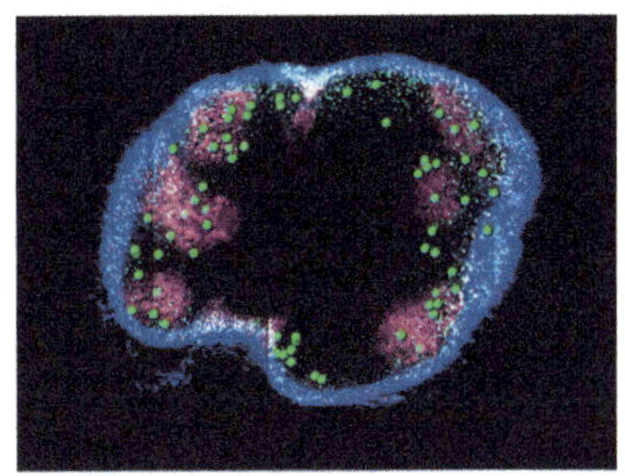

"Memory" B cell (cancer.gov)

For example, the B and T cells that are programmed to seek and destroy the invader we call "measles" are able to destroy *only* measles...or diseases that are very close relatives of measles. The same is true of *all* of the B and T cells in the ranks of the adaptive immune system. These warriors have been programmed to defend the body by engaging a *specific* invader and its close relatives in face-to-face combat (that is, if cells had faces).

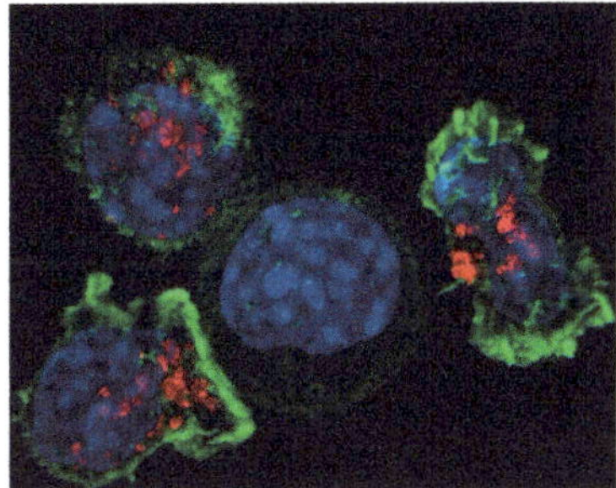

"Killer" T cells surrounding a cancer cell (cancer.gov)

This is how vaccination works. We inject into the body a dose of chemicals that are a miniscule bit of, or else similar to, the disease against which we hope to defend the body. Then we let the adaptive immune system train its B and T defender cells to identify, remember, and kill that specific bit of virus whenever it is detected trying to invade again. And the amazing thing is that *these cells record that lesson for a long time, sometimes for the rest of our lives*, unless they are severely (though rarely) compromised.

The practice of vaccination was most famously and effectively developed in an attempt to ward off the deadly "speckled monster" of human history—smallpox. Although the practice of vaccination as we know it was officially developed by Edward Jenner at the end of the 18th century, there were earlier forms of smallpox vaccination that were practiced in Asia Minor, hundreds of years before Jenner was born. In those earliest treatments (called "variolation"), a drop of fluid from a smallpox patient's pustule was placed under the skin of a non-immune person, who then became immune after being mildly sick. Mildly sick,

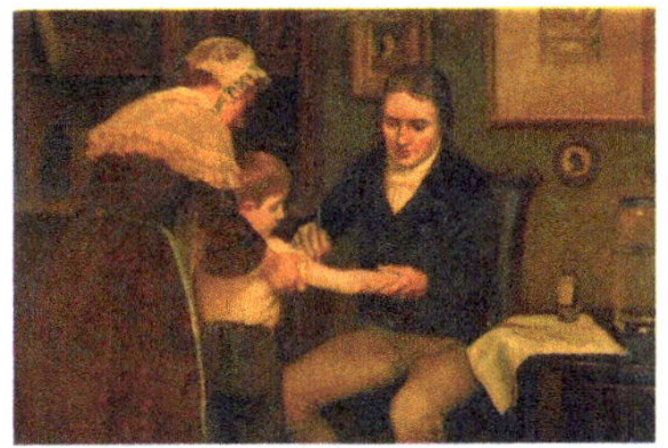

Jenner's first inoculation, Ernest Board (1910) (Wikimedia)

that is, unless that person joined the 2% of variolated patients who contracted a full case of smallpox. But a 2% infection rate was far better than 100%, which is what smallpox could easily inflict on a population, often killing half of them.

As a result of these tiny doses of smallpox being introduced into healthy bodies, the B and T cells in these "variolated" people (as they were then called) were programmed to identify and annihilate any further attempts by *variola major* to invade that person's body. Edward Jenner later discovered that the same immunity to smallpox could be achieved by injecting a small amount of smallpox's close kin—the non-lethal "cowpox" virus—without any danger of the patient developing smallpox from the vaccine. And thus, the practice of safe and widespread vaccination was born.

Unfortunately, the general fear of scientific knowledge, and the particular fear of vaccination, has been with us for centuries, despite the gifts of health and safety that science (and especially vaccination) can afford us. For this reason, Edward Jenner was attacked as well as idolized for his work, even though he was a humble man who directed all proceeds from his discovery to support many humanitarian causes. Fortunately, Jenner was not intimidated by those who feared science and demeaned his work. His devotion to developing his vaccine eventually led to the eradication of smallpox throughout the world by 1980 CE...for the first time in 10,000 years.

And just in case you think this business of developing vaccines is easy, take a look at this list showing the development times for some vaccines that protect us today:

Polio vaccine (1948-1955)—7 years
Measles vaccine (1954-1963)—9 years
Chicken pox vaccine (1954-1988)—34 years
Mumps vaccine (1963-1967)—4 years
HPV vaccine (1991-2006)—15 years
Novel Coronavirus vaccine (2019-2020)—10 months (plus 20 years to develop the mRNA protocol on which it is based)

Once again, it seems crucial to state here that the idea of "herd immunity" may be alluring, but without the medical support afforded only by vaccination, the evolved resistance that some people call "herd immunity" can only reduce the rates of pandemic illness and death from the utterly catastrophic to the merely horrific. Our adaptive immune systems are quick and willing students, but each set of B and T cells in each human body must be given *specific* programming in order to recognize and defeat their *specific* opponent. Without the tiny dose of face-to-face programming that vaccination provides to our B and T cells, the adaptive immune system can do *nothing* to protect us when that deadly invader makes land in our bodies.

Now, along with my apologies for this regrettably simple description of the astonishing complexity that is the human immune system, I will now offer you a brief summary of the ways in which our microscopic defenders have responded to their most deadly opponents throughout human history.

The Immune System versus The Plague

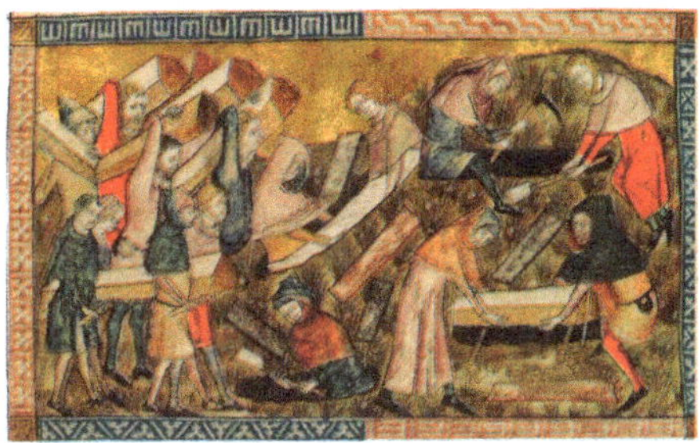

Burying the Dead at Tournai, Pierart dou Tielt (1340-1360) (Wikimedia)

As we learned in the last chapter, there are three forms of plague, in this progressive order of deadliness: bubonic, pneumonic, and septicemic. If plague invades the whole body quickly enough, the immune system cannot mount a defense fast enough to combat it, and the person dies. However, if the plague invasion proceeds more slowly and the person has a robust innate immune system, they *might* survive the infection.

That is why *bubonic* plague is the least lethal of the three types, because it requires several days to infect the body systemically, so the immune system has a chance to mount a defense. Thus, the bubonic plague kills "only" 50 to 60% of its victims. However, once the plague has infected a dense population of humans, it more often presents in its *pneumonic* form, where it is transmitted by exhaled droplets, allowing it to land *first* in the lungs of its next victim. In this pneumonic form, the plague is almost 100% fatal and it kills within one to two days because the body is systemically infected right away, and it has no chance to form an immune defense. Finally, there are rare cases of plague, called *septicemic*, in which the plague bacillus is transmitted directly into the bloodstream. Septicemic plague is almost always lethal and usually kills within a few hours because the body has no time to mount its defense before it becomes fatally septic.

The dramatic interactions between the plague invader *yersinia pestis* and the defenders in the body's immune system are too complex to describe here in purely scientific terms. But if one is willing to trust that metaphor will carry us over an ocean of details, the story of our body's war with plague is surprisingly simple. It begins with the fact that somewhere in the course of plague's millennial history, the bacillus developed an amazing ability (along with that brilliant flea/rat ride-share thing) to sabotage the communication lines of our innate immune system. It does this by injecting a protein called YopJ into some of our immune system's key sentry cells. This act of sabotage prevents the sentries of our immune system from passing the alarm along to the warriors. So, our bodies do not awaken to the threat, nor do they mount a defense, until the plague has fully installed itself in several lymph nodes that have, by this point, exploded with replicating plague bacilli into the excruciating *buboes*. By the time our body realizes that it has been colonized by plague, it must mount a defense so extreme that it usually kills itself while trying to save its life.

What the body attempts to do, in metaphorical terms, is to burn up the infection with its most ferocious incendiary devices, while simultaneously doing other things to prevent its inflammatory fires from burning down the house. Specifically, when the innate immune system finally wakes up to the danger imposed by the plague invaders, it activates a host of cytokine messenger proteins (which you remember because I warned you that they would be important, and now they are, but keep remembering them because they will be important again). For our purposes, it would be accurate to say that the cytokines are released to set off alarms that tell the immune system to 1) incinerate the plague on the one hand, and 2) keep the body from incinerating *itself* on the other. Therefore, these alarm-ringing cytokines fall into two major categories. (And please pay attention here because this part is going to be crucial when we observe how our immune systems react to the novel coronavirus.)

The first cytokines, the ones that ignite the incendiary weapons of immune defense, are called *pro*-inflammatory, and their activation leads to all kinds of biological "fire." Specifically, a *pro*-inflammatory cytokine storm triggers a dilation of the entire circulatory system. Every blood vessel, from the biggest arteries and veins down to the smallest capillaries, expand to maximum capacity in an attempt to flood the body with the red and white blood cells that will super-heat the body, deliver the infection eaters, and destroy the invaders. The resulting symptoms are high fever and the inflammation of tissues and organs. But if this *pro*-inflammatory cytokine storm continues long enough, it will also lead to full-body hemorrhaging and a dangerous loss of blood pressure.

In response to the falling blood pressure and full-body hemorrhaging, the innate immune system unleashes another cytokine storm that sets off its *anti*-inflammatory measures. (The official name for this is CARS, which stands for *compensatory anti-inflammatory response syndrome*, in case you want to impress people at dinner parties. Assuming we ever get to have impressive dinner parties again.) In CARS, the *anti*-inflammatory cytokines trigger the *constriction* of all the blood vessels and induce body-wide blood-clotting (also called "coagulation" or "thrombosis"), which is meant to stop the hemorrhaging. The formal name for this extreme situation is *disseminated intravascular coagulation* (DIC), and it is important to remember because we're going to meet it again when we return to the war that our immune systems will be waging with the coronavirus.

In simple terms, this second cytokine cascade is trying to cool the waters and plug the leaks that were started by the inflammatory firestorm. Unfortunately, the DIC creates a blizzard of tiny clots throughout the circulatory system, often plugging blood flow to our vital organs. And that causes our vital organs to malfunction and eventually shut down. This shutdown, as you can imagine, is *seriously* bad news for the body's survival. Indeed, this event is called "multi-organ failure," and I don't think I have to say much more to convey how lethal it is. One organ after another—liver, kidneys, lungs, heart, brain—surrenders to a deadly darkness.

To repeat, the innate immune system wages this two-pronged attack in a desperate war for the body's survival by 1) activating its pro-inflammatory measures to burn up the invader, and 2) activating anti-inflammatory countermeasures to keep from burning up itself in the process. This simultaneous flood of pro- and anti-inflammatory messages has sometimes been called "competing cytokine storms," although in a rare moment of poetic inspiration, one immunologist dubbed it "thrombo-hemorrhagic derangement." This compelling term implies that the body's immune defenders have driven the vascular system completely insane with their conflicting efforts to use both bleeding and clotting to kill the disease invaders while preserving the body that's being invaded.

These shifts—from the immune system's initial firefight, to its competing tactics of pro- and anti-inflammation, to its final state of clot-induced organ failure—are what immunologists refer to as "a transition from *systemic inflammatory response* (SIRS) to *septic shock*." Rarely do we survive once our bodies have entered the state of septic shock. It is the tragic moment when a desperately fought battle against the invader turns against the defenders and they are slaughtered by the weapons of their own defense. It is what happens when our innate immune system's frantic efforts to save us finally descend into a catastrophic collision of bleeding (hemorrhage) and clotting (thrombosis). In the midst of this biochemical chaos, and in the face of an undefeated invader, our overwhelmed body quite reasonably surrenders to the maelstrom and dies.

The Immune System versus Smallpox

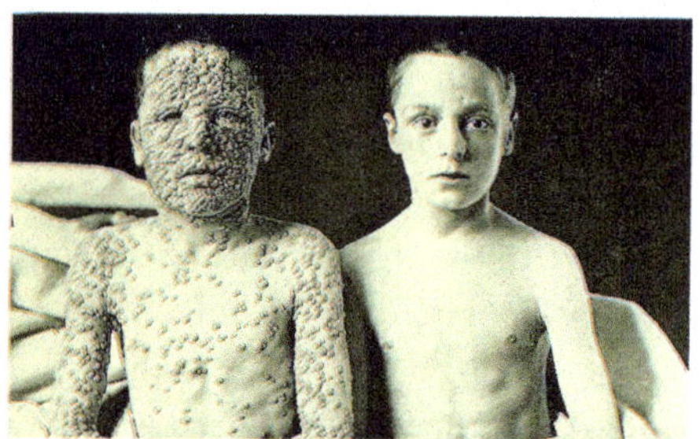

Smallpox—unvaccinated versus vaccinated (1901)
(The Jenner Trust) (Wikimedia)

We now know a great deal about the virus *variola major* that was responsible for smallpox, in the sense that we understand its structure, manifestation, and means of transmission. However, it is still unknown exactly how, biologically, smallpox led to the death of its victims. We do know that the virus could prevent the production of interferon, which protects us by preventing a virus from replicating.[33] But as for the actual cause of death, we can only say that it appears from historical accounts that the body of a smallpox victim finally succumbed to multiple organ failure, probably due to "uncontrolled immune response."[34]

Initially, the smallpox virus dodges the immune system by releasing a protein that deactivates one of the innate immune system's primary weapons,

33. del Mar, Fernandez de Marco. "The highly virulent variola and monkeypox viruses express secreted inhibitors of type I interferon." *The FASEB Journal*, 2009. DOI: 10.1096/fj.09-144733

34. Atkinson William, Jennifer Hamborsky, Lynne McIntyre and Charles (Skip) Wolfe, eds. "Smallpox" in *Epidemiology and Prevention of Vaccine-Preventable Diseases (The Pink Book)* (9th ed.). Washington DC: Public Health Foundation, 2005, pp. 281–306. https://stacks.cdc.gov/view/cdc/78725/cdc_78725_DS1.pdf

interferon. Similar to the progress of a plague infection, by the time the body awakens to the threat, it is often too late to incinerate the invaders without burning down the house they have invaded.

Once the innate immune system is triggered by the smallpox infection, it responds with what appears to some immunologists (based on historical accounts) to be a cytokine storm like the one that occurs in third-degree burn victims. In other words, the cytokines ignite a massive inflammatory process throughout the body to combat the smallpox infection as it spreads, and the effects of that storm continue to cascade unabated. Blood and serum gush to the extremities, filling them with white blood cells in an apparent attempt to boil the infected tissues clean with the body's equivalent of hot water.

Meanwhile, the *variola* virus progressively dries out every organ, especially the body's protective container of skin (which is an organ, too). In the end, a body infected with smallpox almost literally burns up, both from its own inflammatory heat and from the viral desiccation. And given how the innate immune system works, we can assume it eventually unleashes its secondary anti-inflammatory cytokine storm, triggering the systemic clotting that leads to multiple organ failure and septic shock.

This description of our immune response to smallpox is derived from 20th century case files, but it corresponds to ancient descriptions of smallpox patients written by historical physicians and reported in C.W. Dixon's landmark book, *Smallpox*:

> Jenulf, writing in 923 CE, said: "It is shocking to hear the groans of the sufferers, to see parts of their bodies as if burnt, dissolving away, and to smell the intolerable foetor of their putrid flesh." And in 944 CE, "pestilence of fire occurred in Limosila, where innumerable bodies of men and women were consumed by visible fire, and also in Aquitaine." And in the 11th century CE, "the people died miserably from their limbs being burnt black from a sacred fire."[35]

In the throes of this biochemical firestorm, the exhausted body would die in the clutches of the dreaded "pox." Or if the body lived, it bore forever the physical and emotional scarring that makes the smallpox invader such a horrifying medical monster, even to our modern eyes.

35. Dixon, Cyril William. *Smallpox*. London: J. & A. Churchill, 1962, p. 188.

The Immune System versus the 1918 Flu

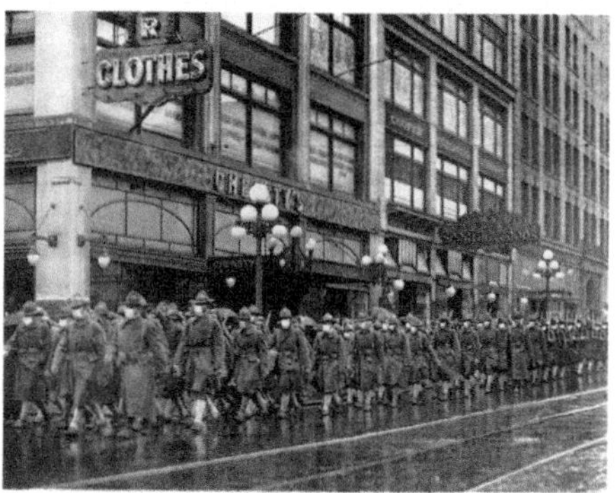

American soldiers marching to transport ships in 1918...

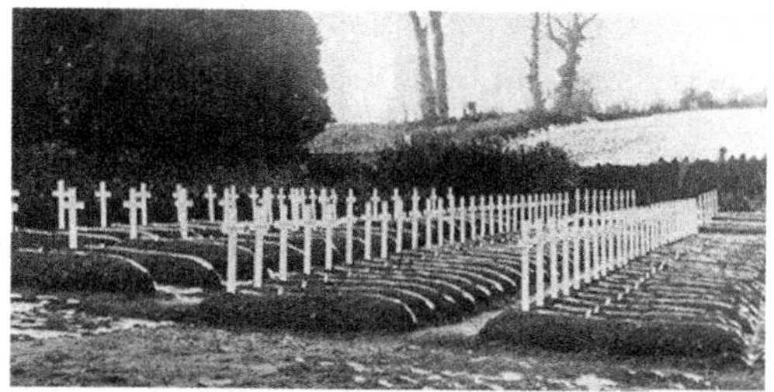

...and those who became flu victims later in the year.
(Wikimedia)

First observed in March 1918, *influenza H1N1* began as only a moderate monster, and not the deadly scourge it would eventually become. It traveled with the American soldiers to World War I, where it was finally mentioned by the war-neutral Spanish press, and *only* the Spanish press, thereby acquiring (very unfairly) its original name—"the Spanish flu." As mentioned in the previous chapter, the virus mutated over the next few months such that it began its real killing spree in August 1918.

Previously, *influenza H1N1* had behaved as all flu viruses had behaved before 1918, precipitating fever, aches, and severe respiratory symptoms. However, after the virus returned in the summer of 1918, traveling to the United States and other parts of the world with the furloughed troops, the character of its symptoms changed. Some people still manifested the traditional flu pattern, but many people, especially those of robust health aged 25 to 35, were known to die of respiratory failure within a day or two, and sometimes within a few hours.

Viewed through the lenses of modern immunology, it seems that the second wave of the 1918 flu pandemic precipitated a cytokine storm that was only *pro*-inflammatory in these robust young people. In autopsies performed at the time, it was documented that their otherwise healthy lungs were filled with fluid containing red and white blood cells. The modern interpretation of these cases is that a pro-inflammatory cytokine storm ignited a flood of white and red cells in the person's lungs, apparently the result of the innate immune system's excessive attempt to combat this deadly respiratory virus.

The body's immune response was heroic, but its tactics were lethally overzealous. For whatever reason, the body could not reduce or counteract its cascade of *pro*-inflammatory cytokines, leaving the flu-infected person to drown in the fluids of their own immune response...or else succumb to the secondary bacterial pneumonias that often proliferated in fluid-filled lungs during this pre-antibiotic age. Once again, it was not the invading protagonist that directly killed its victims in 1918; it was the overblown response of the body's immune antagonists.

The Immune System versus The Novel Coronavirus

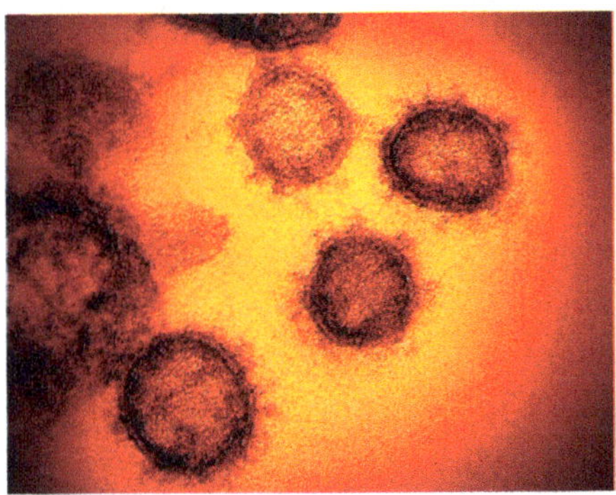

Electron microscopic photo of *novel coronavirus*, 370K magnification (NIAID)

So now we have this novel coronavirus, which appears to have our immune systems completely flummoxed. Or at least that's what happens in *some* bodies. And that's one of the things that is both mesmerizing and horrifying about this story.

Let's start with the fact that this virus—like plague, smallpox, and influenza H1N1—is a gift from our animal cousins. Well, that's true of most serious diseases. This is why the Native American populations were decimated after the arrival of Europeans in the 15th century ; they had never maintained daily close contact with animals, as the Old World peoples had done for millennia in the course of domesticating various species. But let's be clear here. What is currently being referred to as the "herd immunity" of the Old World inhabitants was more like evolved resistance; *it still included a child mortality rate of more than 40%.* (Yes, believe it. At least four out of ten children in 15th century Europe died before adulthood.) But the Old World heritage of animal husbandry did give its populations *some* advantage, as did the fact that the Europeans who arrived in the New World were among the 60% who had survived the childhood ravages of the Old World's endemic diseases.

The New World inhabitants, on the other hand, were *not* the descendants of countless generations who had tended domestic animals and survived the myriad diseases they shared, nor had they survived a host of endemic diseases in their own childhoods, as the Europeans had. Thus, the immune systems of the New World inhabitants had *no* capacity to repel, or even mitigate, the onslaught of new bacteria and viruses that were carried in the bodies and belongings of the conquistadores. And as a result, nearly all those defenseless indigenous bodies died in the multiple waves of epidemic disease that burned across the American continents during the century following Columbus's arrival.

Of course, it's been several centuries since the pandemic holocaust of the post-Columbian Americas, and most human immune systems—our coordinated armies of micro-defenders—have either evolved or been carefully programmed by vaccination to defend us against the worst of our pandemic invaders. But despite all that, there is something about the novel coronavirus that is enabling it to spread like wildfire and scorch our species today. Thankfully, this is no longer a complete mystery. It turns out that we can understand much about the character of our current invader by observing how our immune systems respond to its campaign of colonization. In fact, the behaviors of our body's defenders initially told us more about the nature of the novel coronavirus than what we could directly learn from the virus itself.

It's rather like what happened when astronomers were trying to identify the celestial body that we call Pluto. For many years, astronomers did not have telescopes powerful enough to see Pluto directly, but they *knew* it was there because they could clearly detect the ways in which Pluto was distorting the flight paths of asteroids and comets and even planets that passed within its gravitational field. Similarly, the novel coronavirus has revealed much about its essential nature by the way in which it is distorting the conduct of our immune systems and our bodies.[36]

Consider, for example, the fact that the virus was originally labeled as a "respiratory disease" because its first symptoms are often respiratory symptoms. And indeed, we have since learned that the novel coronavirus is, in fact, primarily transmitted via airborne means—"aerosol" droplets suspended in the air for prolonged periods of time. But many scientists had already assumed that the coronavirus was airborne because of its transmission speed. Blood-borne viruses like HIV simply can't spread that fast.

In the end, however, it was Covid-19's 1) *variability of symptoms* that physicians observed over time, and 2) *the wide variety of body parts* in which its symptoms were observed, that strongly suggested the novel coronavirus was *not* primarily a respiratory virus, because it didn't remain in the respiratory system for replication. (Remember? Viruses only locate places to replicate...and then they replicate. Nothing more.)

Now we know that novel coronavirus replicates in the ACE2 receptors, meaning that it can travel and make camp wherever ACE2 receptors are most plentiful...meaning the entire vascular system. And that makes this coronavirus a *vascular* disease, rather than a respiratory disease. The ability of coronavirus to bond and replicate in the ACE2 receptors enables it to proliferate throughout our blood vessels and in most of our vital organs (kidneys, liver, gut, brain, and heart, as well as lungs), because those are all places where ACE2 receptors abound. We did eventually learn about that ACE2 receptor business by direct observation, but even before that evidence was secured, scientists were already deducing something like it from the Covid-induced patterns in our symptoms and immune responses. This viral Pluto revealed itself through its effects, long before we could observe it directly.

Similarly, it has not required microscopic evidence for scientists and physicians to know that our innate immune systems are frequently baffled by this beast. The virologists understood this pretty quickly because of the diverse ways in which Covid-19 manifests in different bodies, and the diverse ways in which the immune systems of different bodies are trying to combat it...with diverse results:

36. For the following discussion, I am beholden to the very excellent (albeit early) review article entitled "How does coronavirus kill? Clinicians trace a ferocious rampage through the body, from brain to toes," by Meredith Wadman, Jennifer Couzin-Frankel, Jocelyn Kaiser, and Catherine Matacic in *Science*, April 17, 2020. https://www.science.org/content/article/how-does-coronavirus-kill-clinicians-trace-ferocious-rampage-through-body-brain-toes

1. Some immune systems seem to wave off the virus like a fly, showing no symptoms at all, even though serology tests show that a Covid-19 infection has occurred. (And of course, some of these folks suffered hidden damage that only showed up later).
2. Other immune systems succumb rapidly and proceed directly to death, with nary a sign of immune response (no fever, no struggle, etc.). It's as if these immune systems have no idea what to do with this beast, nor even that their bodies have been invaded.
3. Still other immune systems fight the virus ferociously, based on the body's severe symptoms, and appear to fight it off. But then it comes back, so they fight it off again, and then it comes back again, and so it goes for weeks.
4. And still other immune systems show little sign of a struggle… until the body manifests catastrophic clotting storms that are now being documented in younger, healthy people around the world. This is rather like the second wave of the 1918 flu—a situation that looks as if the immune system is switching on, but is unable to switch off before injuring or killing its own body.

We also know the novel coronavirus is confounding our immune systems because of the wide range of *locations* in the human body that it can infect, often unchallenged. This invader has laid claim to a *huge* variety of campsites, because these are all the places where ACE2 receptors are located, including:

Nasal cells	Eyes	Kidney	Prostate	Lungs	Liver
Pancreas	Testicles	Heart	Bladder	Brain	Placenta
Adipose cells [37]					

This tells us that novel coronavirus is able to move freely and set up camp widely in any body whose immune system cannot quickly muster an effective defense against the invader.[38] And we have recently learned that

37. Yes, that would be *fat cells*. In other words, the more fat you have, the more coronavirus replication sites you have. Which seems terribly unjust to me. But then again, no one asked my opinion. (See Saccon, Tatiana Dandolini, Felippe Mousovich-Neto, Riassa Guimarães Ludwig, *et al.* "SARS-CoV-2 infects adipose tissue in a fat depot- and viral lineage-dependent manner." *Nature Communications*, 13, 5722 (September 29, 2022). https://doi.org/10.1038/s41467-022-33218-8

38. Baraniuk, Chris. "Receptors for SARS-CoV-2 Present in Wide Variety of Human Cells." *The Scientist*, April 29, 2020. https://www.the-scientist.com/news-opinion/receptors-for-sars-cov-2-present-in-wide-variety-of-human-cells-67496

SARS CoV-2 can have enduring effects on our blood's clotting chemistry and our body's immunizing molecules such that both can be seriously compromised into the syndrome we now call "long Covid."[39]

These wide ranges of symptom presentations, disease progressions, and recuperation outcomes tell us that novel coronavirus is unlike all of the other protagonists we have met in humanity's pandemic history. Certainly, individual people always differ in the way they respond to a microscopic invader. But none of our other pandemic killers—not plague, not smallpox, and not H1N1 flu—have ever produced such a diverse set of symptoms, progressions, and outcomes.

Metaphorically speaking, we could say that plague, smallpox, and H1N1 each developed specific talents that have enabled them to colonize and conquer millions of humans around the world over many years. But each of these diseases only shows one or two special talents—a mode of interspecies transport (like plague), or a means of initially dodging the immune system in order to set up a base camp (like plague and smallpox), or the ignition of excessive immune response (like H1N1), and so forth.

The novel coronavirus is, by contrast, a viral pentathlete. It has a *host* of special talents, the sum of which gives it a unique advantage when placed in combat against the human immune system. We saw the following list in the last chapter, but let's take a quick look at it again in summary. Novel coronavirus is:

1. Highly contagious.
2. Not highly lethal, so it can move to a new population before killing all its hosts.
3. Slow to show symptoms, so the host is contagious long before knowing it.
4. Establishes replication sites in a wide range of body organs.
5. Becomes and remains contagious at indeterminate times.
6. Does not confer full immunity through the adaptive immune system.
7. Circulates in "swarms" of differing strains, as well as mutating to new forms.

39. Turner, Simone, Caitlin A. Naidoo, Thomas J. Usher, Arneaux Kruger, Chantelle Venter, Gert Jacobus Laubscher, M. Asad Khan, Douglas B. Kell and Etherasia Pretorius. "Increased levels of inflammatory molecules in blood of Long COVID patients point to thrombotic endotheliitis." *medRxiv*, October 18, 2022. https://www.medrxiv.org/content/10.1101/2022.10.13.22281055v1

No other pandemic protagonist has ever possessed all of these advantages together. This makes the novel coronavirus a daunting opponent to our defending immune systems. And that's exactly what we're seeing in the effects that the virus is having on the behavior of our immune systems and bodies over time. This is a powerful and dangerously influential "Pluto," judging by the myriad ways it is distorting our immune responses and our bodies' symptoms.

Of course, we are finally acquiring a few direct views of our viral Pluto after several years of combatting it. For example, we now know about that ACE2 access business, which was crucial in the development of a vaccine. For the moment, however, we must rely much more on what we can observe in the behaviors of our defending immune systems, and the symptoms in our faithful bodies, in order to profile this lethal invader. The variety of symptoms, severities, progressions, and prognoses that are ignited by novel coronavirus are astounding for *any* disease, but especially when compared to the ways our internal defenders have responded to the other invaders that we have met in pandemic history. Every deadly pandemic disease has confounded our immune systems in one way or another, but *no other major pandemic disease has ever invaded the human body so variably, nor confounded its immune system so diversely.*

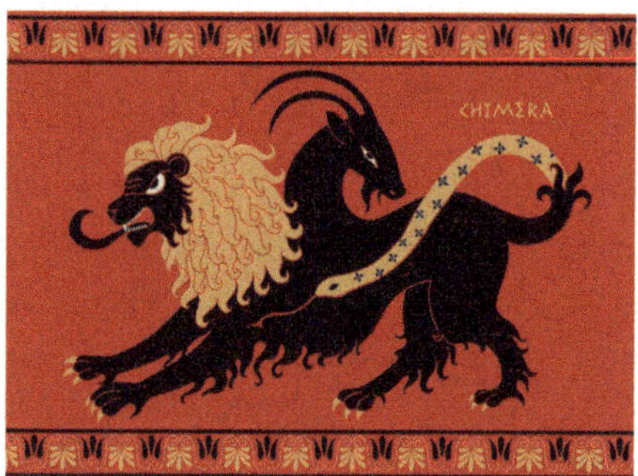

The Chimera, depicted in the style of ancient Greece (Shutterstock)

Viewed from the perspective of our defending immune armies, the threat posed by Covid-19 evokes a terrifying myth from ancient Greece—the multiply-menacing *Chimera*. The historian/poet Hesiod describes the Chimera as, "A creature fearsome, great, swift-footed and strong, who had three heads—one of a grim-eyed lion, another of a goat, and another of a snake or fierce dragon; in her forepart she was a lion; in her hinderpart, a dragon; and in her middle, a goat, breathing forth a fearful blast of blazing fire."[40] The Chimera was a terrifying enemy to all living things, and she was reputed to have bred other monsters as dangerous as

40. Hesiod. "The Homeric Hymns and Homerica." *Theogony 325*. Translated by Hugh G. Evelyn-White. Cambridge, MA: Harvard University Press, 1914.

herself, including the deadly Sphinx who mythically challenged Oedipus and who still guards the Egyptian pyramids.

Although the name Chimera was originally used to describe this terrifying mythic creature of multiple lethality, the label has come to denote any creature, mythic or actual, that is a conglomerate being. The man/horse creature that we call "centaur" is a mythical chimera. The horse/donkey offspring that we call "mule" is a biological chimera. There are even instances in which one animal, including a human animal, can become a chimera by carrying two sets of DNA—for example, as the result of absorbing one's nonviable twin *in utero*, or as the consequence of an organ transplant.

There has been a hotly debated proposal that the novel coronavirus is a "chimera virus"—a hybrid of two other viruses.[41] There are insufficient data to say anything conclusive about that proposal at this moment, so let's focus on the undeniable fact that the novel coronavirus poses a threat that is *metaphorically* similar to the multiple threats that the mythic Chimera posed to her victims. She was exceptionally dangerous because each of her three aspects—lion, wild goat, and dragon—possessed the fighting talent of its individual nature. In addition, the Chimera could breathe fire, which made her utterly invincible...until the hero Bellerophon arrived, mounted on his winged horse Pegasus.

Because Bellerophon and Pegasus could leap beyond the Chimera's attack range (she didn't have wings, thank the gods), they could escape the worst of her weapons while launching their own assaults. In the end, Bellerophon charged Pegasus directly at the Chimera and rammed a lump of lead down the throat of her fire-breathing ram portion, stoppering her flame and suffocating the beast until she died.

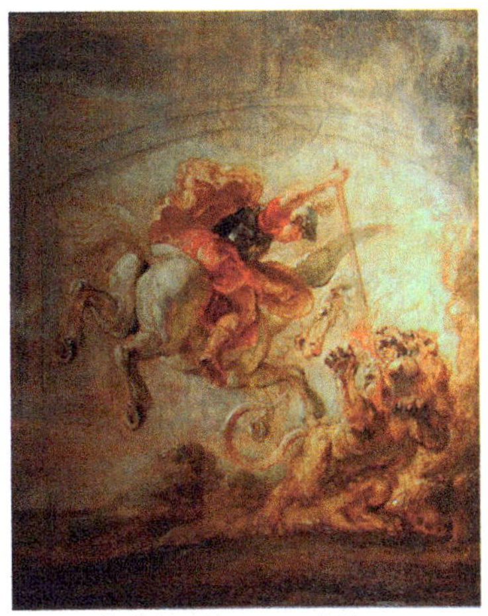

Bellerophon, Pegasus and Chimera,
Peter Paul Rubens, 1635
(Wikimedia)

Whether or not the novel coronavirus is literally a "chimera virus," there is value in the metaphor that the Chimera myth offers us, especially as we consider the battle we are waging

41. Wade, Nicolas. "The origin of COVID: Did people or nature open Pandora's box at Wuhan?" *Bulletin of the Atomic Scientists*, May 5, 2021. https://thebulletin.org/2021/05/the-origin-of-covid-did-people-or-nature-open-pandoras-box-at-wuhan/

with this lethal invader in the current pandemic. Let us imagine that the investigators who followed in the wake of the mythic Chimera could only deduce her nature and weapons from the damage she inflicted and the destruction she left behind. This retrospective kind of detective work has been our strategy with every pandemic invader we have ever faced, especially before we could see bacteria and viruses with our microscopes. We developed each disease's murderous "profile" based on its pattern of invasion and destruction.

Of course, with our most lethal invaders, we have at least been able to find *consistent* evidence of the battle between the invading disease and the defenders in our innate immune system. For example, a person could set their watch by the progression of smallpox in its victims. Consistent symptom sets like that have enabled us to paint a fairly clear portrait of the invader we were fighting. And until very recently, a disease's "symptom portrait" was almost all we had to out-maneuver our pandemic opponent.

But with the novel coronavirus, we have faced the same challenge that the mythic investigators faced when they surveyed the wreckage left by the Chimera—that is, we saw many kinds of damage, initially indicating several kinds of perpetrator. We can imagine those ancient investigators asking themselves, "Is this killer a dragon? Or a ram? Or a lion?" And finally, "What the hell *is* this murderous beast?" Similarly, the scientists and physicians in 2020 began by asking, "Is this a disease of the respiratory system? The kidneys? The liver? The gut? The brain? The immune system? How does this virus attack, injure, and kill? What the hell *is* this murderous beast?"

In the end, the same beast—novel coronavirus—is inflicting *all* sorts of damage, inciting our immune systems to malfunction in many ways. In the past, we have battled one pandemic beast at a time—the lion of plague, the ram of flu, the dragon of smallpox. *This* time, we are facing a pandemic chimera. *This* time, we need special weapons, special allies, and special skills beyond those of our faithful our immunological defenders. *This* time, we must call in the Larger Forces, as did the folks in the ancient Chimera myth, in order to defeat the beast.

It is time to turn to the second group of defenders in our story, the defenders whose tactics are larger, slower, and initially more cumbersome than the blazingly elegant weapons of the human immune system. But when you are facing a pandemic invader of unprecedented talents and variability (and here again, that word "unprecedented" is well justified), you must call upon the heroic elements of human courage and intelligence to rise on the wings of human creativity in order to develop complex defensive tactics, culminating in a vaccine that can program the assassins of humanity's adaptive immune system to stopper the beast.

Time to meet the large-scale defenders of our story, some whose efforts will save our species, and some whose misguided efforts will serve to threaten the entire campaign for human survival.

Time to meet the human race...

CHAPTER 4

Finally, Let's Meet Our Bravest Defenders in Any Pandemic

Humanity versus Pestilence—Macro-Defenders versus Micro-Invaders

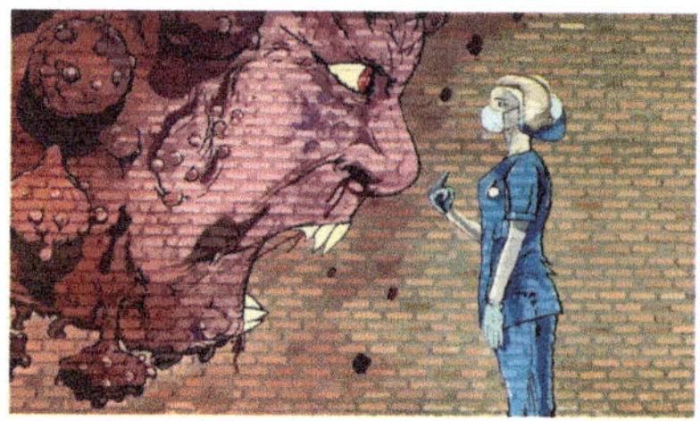

Graffiti in the Srinakarin train station, Thailand, May 2020 (Shutterstock)

Cowards die many times before their deaths;
The valiant never taste of death but once.
– William Shakespeare, *Julius Caesar*, II.ii

Do not go gentle into that good night.
Rage, rage against the dying of the light.
– Dylan Thomas[42]

Since the dawn of time, pandemic disease has attacked and annihilated countless species on the Earth. Humankind is the only species that has ever dared to fight back.

There is something astonishing in this fact, not only because we are unique in our biological audacity, but also because we are a very *vulnerable* species, especially when compared to many others. Yes, we have large brains and some remarkable adaptive abilities. But we also possess a host of frailties that make us fertile ground for aspiring microbes, including the deadly microbes that we've met in this book. Not all species are as vulnerable to disease as we are.

Consider, for example, that many of the deadly pathogens that have

42. Thomas, Dylan. "Do not go gentle into that good night." *The Poems of Dylan Thomas.* New York, NY: New Directions, 1947/2017, 239. Copyright © 1952 by Dylan Thomas. Reprinted by permission of New Directions Publishing Corporation.

afflicted our species—including the SARS, MERS, Ebola, and Marburg viruses, as well as the SARS CoV-2 virus—have come to us from *bats*. And all of these viruses live peacefully in the bodies of *healthy* bats, without igniting any notable bat diseases.

Scientists have concluded that this is because the immune systems of bats are much less sensitive than ours, much less prone to the cytokine storms and inflammatory cascades that we learned about in the last chapter. This, it seems, is because bats *fly*, and the metabolic changes that are required to go from zero to airborne would incinerate bats if their immune systems were as sensitive as ours. So, the immune systems of bats are comparatively dull and sluggish, and that's why bats are tolerant to many viruses that become deadly when attacked by our hyper-reactive human immune systems.[43]

Despite our vulnerable bodies, or perhaps because of them, we humans have uniquely refused to go gentle into the not-so-good night of pandemic disease. And we have been digging our collective heels into the quicksand of pandemic survival since long before we had any factual notions about the *causes* for our deadly diseases. We simply fought back as best we could. Only us. Panic-stricken as we were.

To get a sense of the terror that pandemic diseases have ignited in us, we need only look at the Bible's book of Revelation, which offers one of the most compelling and enduring images of human demise: The Four Horsemen of the Apocalypse. The order of the Horsemen's appearance in that dream-like narrative is the following:

1. **Pestilence** is mounted on a white horse,
2. **War** is riding a red horse,

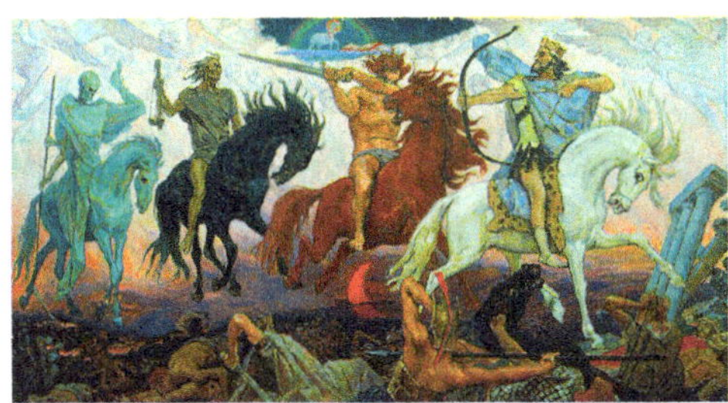

Four Horsemen of the Apocalypse, Victor Vasnetsov (1887) (Wikimedia)

43. Ehrenberg, Rachel. "Why do bats have so many viruses?" *The Washington Post,* July 15, 2020. https://www.washingtonpost.com/science/why-do-bats-have-so-many-viruses/2020/07/10/0327f584-b65e-11ea-a8da-693df3d7674a_story.html

3. **Famine** is on a black horse, and
4. **Death** is on the infamous "pale" horse…which is technically a corpse-like green (yes, green).

From the perspective of Jungian psychology, there are no random details in any symbol or myth. Thus, it is no accident that the *first* of the apocalyptic equestrians is…Pestilence. Evidently, even the ancients considered pandemic disease to be a supremely horrifying killer. As Albert Camus observed in his landmark novel *The Plague* (*La Peste*), "A pestilence isn't a thing made to man's measure."[44]

Our species has always been confounded by the superhuman dimensions of pandemic disease. To quote Camus again, "There have been as many plagues as wars in history; yet plagues and wars always take people equally by surprise."[45] It's as if we cannot hold in consciousness the lethal potential of our fellow humans, nor the vastly *more* lethal power of our microscopic invaders. But the real surprise is that, unlike humanity's apparent acceptance of war, famine, and random mischance as the dealers of death, we humans have made some truly heroic efforts to combat the scourge of pestilence. No other species has ever attempted that.

This is not to say, of course, that our species has ever achieved wide consensus or resounding success when we have opposed our pandemic diseases, and certainly not while those infectious invaders were actively assaulting us. Indeed, our human behaviors have historically achieved much *less* success than what has been achieved by our microscopic allies in the human immune system.

But our efforts as defenders of our bodies have been noteworthy enough to bear examination in this book. Against all odds, we macro-defenders have, somewhat surprisingly, achieved *enough* success against our micro-invaders to merit respect, if only because we have *chosen* to fight…unlike our immune systems, which have no choice but to fight, and unlike all the other species, which have never exercised whatever defensive choices they may have had.

So, let's see what kinds of war we have waged against Pestilence…

♦ ♦ ♦

44. Camus, Albert. *The Plague (La Peste)*. Translated by Stuart Gilbert. New York, NY: Vintage, 1948/1975, 37.

45. Ibid, p. 38

This will be a story filled with heroism and foolishness, audacity and cowardice, inspiration and idiocy. It is a *human* story, after all, which means it is a story about a group of unlikely creatures who crawled out of the savannah, slowly stood upright, and eventually looked at the sky. We are the creatures who not only had an ability to *see* the stars, but to wonder what those stars might *be*.[46] We are the creatures whose relative frailty has been largely defended by our capacity to *learn* things...often some truly amazing things that were *well* beyond what was necessary for our survival.

Indeed, for the entirety of our existence, we humans have been dancing the stressful tightrope, described so well by Friedrich Nietzsche, that is suspended between our animal realities and our transcendent possibilities.[47] This tightrope recalls the stressful tension that hums between our competing needs for familiarity vs. novelty, comfort vs. adventure, predictability vs. mystery. The ways in which each of us responds to these stressors, and the ways in which each of us even *defines* a stressor, are related to the unique ways in which each of us dances on the Nietzschean tightrope—dances between the world of matter and the world of mind, between what is mortally finite and what is deathlessly infinite, between what is known and what is still unknown. One person's titillation is another person's trauma. This is the dark humor of the human stress response repertoire.

Of course, pandemics are painfully stressful for *everyone*, by definition. Death, disease, and suffering on a massive scale cannot be otherwise. But individual animals, including individual human animals, have always displayed a wide variety of responses to stress, including pandemic-induced stress. And that is what we find when we look at the human defenders in the stories of pandemics...including the coronavirus pandemic. So let's see what different kinds of stress response we find when we take that look.

What are the Different Ways We Respond to Stress, Pandemic Stress Included?

One of the hardest tasks for humankind is to balance our life-preserving need to make accurate predictions against our sanity-preserving desire to ignore terrible news.

46. And even more unbelievably, creatures who have recently launched a telescope that shows us 13 billion-year-old light from the origins of those stars.

47. Nietzsche, Friedrich. *Thus Spoke Zarathustra*, translated by R. J. Hollingdale. Harmondsworth: Penguin Books, 1883–1885/1961.

Not that we are such great predictors under the happiest of circumstances. The tidal wave of information that continually sweeps over us is vastly greater than our thimble-sized capacity to reduce it into precise predictions. Or do you believe that weather forecasts, scientific as they are, will be perfect? Now, compare the stream of scientific information that we use to create weather forecasts against the waves of emotionally-charged information that pour over us every single minute. Clearly, it's a miracle that we can predict what we're going to have for breakfast, let alone how we're going to survive a global pandemic.

Well, the fact is that we *don't* usually predict what we're going to have for breakfast, because we dump most of life's complexity into the categories of Habits, Assumptions, and Stuff We Ignore. And when we *do* make predictions, we rely on a variety of quick-and-dirty shortcuts that psychologists call *heuristics*—the non-logical, instantaneous, and unconscious tactics that we employ to reach most of our conclusions.

Heuristics can produce conclusions that range from the surprisingly accurate (given their lack of solid data) to the certifiably lunatic (although the person who depends on them rarely sees them that way). But rather like the innate immune system, heuristics are essential to our ability to function in the world because their predictions are fast and furious—"furious" in that they carry the clout of *emotional certainty*. Heuristic conclusions are always biased and often erroneous, but who's got time to mess with logic and truth when a rapid response is required? The conclusions that heuristics produce serve to reassure us and propel us forward in life, and that's why we rely on them for most of our decision-making, even in the cases where they are literally, and sometimes lethally, false.

Vast amounts of research in the second half of the 20th century were devoted to identifying the different kinds of heuristics that we use to make judgements and predictions. [48] Most of that research seemed to demonstrate that although we rely on heuristics that are *occasionally* accurate (albeit quirky), in most cases, our heuristic "logic" is simply laughable. It makes you wonder how we have survived through all these millennia, relying on such wonky strategies as random timing, biased sampling, gut feelings, and unfounded beliefs. Indeed, the heuristics research makes it sound as if humankind has been charting its way through life armed with nothing more than a comic book, a box of crayons, and dumb luck. And maybe that's the truth.

48. For one excellent example: Kahneman, Daniel, Paul Slovic, and Amos Tversky. *Judgement Under Uncertainty: Heuristics and Biases.* New York: Cambridge University Press, 1982.

It is certainly the truth that most human animals have responded to the challenges of reacting to pandemics in the same way that most non-human animals have. That is, most of us have simply suffered and died in the microscopic clutches of our pandemic invaders—mindlessly, horrifically, and voluminously. But sometimes we humans have *not* succumbed to pestilence with mute anguish and blind despair. Sometimes we have tried to outwit our mysterious attackers and we fought back. And in some cases, to some degree, we have succeeded. Let's see which human behaviors have propelled us to those successes…and which behaviors have led us to much more regrettable ends.

Meeting Our Human Stress Responses [49]

I mentioned earlier that every pandemic must inevitably involve stress. And we're talking about *extreme* stress for most people when those micro-invaders colonize our bodies, because pandemics bring death on a scale that is far more horrifying than any other lethal force known to our species. More horrifying, and often more mysterious, which makes pandemics even more frightening than most things that kill us. Bacteria and viruses have been invisible for most of human history, of course, but pandemics continue to be terrifying, even to our modern selves, because of the eerie workings of contagion, mutation, and plain dumb luck (bad and good). Which you probably know yourself after spending years playing stress-tag with the novel coronavirus.

There is a great variety in the ways that human beings respond to stress, and each form of response will determine what the human defender will or won't be able to accomplish when confronting that pandemic invader. For the most part, we will see that a person's style of responding to stress will tell us what *kind* of pandemic defender that person is likely to be—productive, counterproductive, or innocuous. And this business of stress response styles will bring us back to the business of heuristics. Sort of. Well,

49. The psychologically initiated among you will recognize that these "stress responses" bear a strong resemblance to the behavior patterns that Sigmund Freud called "defense mechanisms," and subsequent psychologists more euphemistically called "coping strategies." But many current psychologists prefer the term "stress responses" because Freud's label of "defense mechanism" implies a position of innate opposition (i.e. defensiveness) that is not applicable to all these responses. And "coping strategies" implies that all of these responses entail some level of coping and/or some level of strategizing...neither of which is true for many of them. Thus, the majority of us have settled upon "stress responses," because they are all identifiable patterns of response to an infinite variety of stressors. So there.

anyway, they're related. In general, we can say that our stress responses fall into three broad categories:

1. Stress responses with mostly helpful consequences,
2. Stress responses with unpredictable or neutral consequences, and
3. Stress responses with consequences that almost *never* turn out well.

Now, just because some people depend on the stress responses that almost never turn out well, that doesn't mean they will stop using them. You see, *the reasons that we tend to employ a certain stress response depend far more on* ***emotions*** *than on logic. And the emotional reasons that motivate some of us to select particular stress responses also motivate us to* ***cling*** *to them, even if those responses repeatedly lead us into trouble.*

During the coronavirus pandemic, for example, much has been written about why some people stubbornly reject certain behaviors—such as mask-wearing and social distancing—that have been proven to reduce Covid contagion and death. The three culprits most responsible for these destructive choices are the heuristics that psychologists call "intolerance for ambiguity,"[50] "reduction of cognitive dissonance,"[51] and "confirmation sampling bias."[52] These three behavioral quirks are driven, respectively, by our search for simplicity, reason, and reassurance in a world that is filled with complexity, contradictions, and risk. Or during a lethal pandemic, extreme danger.

Of course, no matter how educated and rational we believe ourselves to be, nearly all of us prefer world views that offer comforting and coherent explanations for the things we see. In other words, we prefer a "consonant" view of the world, because that gives us the feeling that we can predict and manage the whirlwind that is Life. If the world starts to feel too "dissonant"—too discordant, too irrational, too contradictory—we get worried that we will be lost in the chaos.

For some of us, the dissonance of the world hits a level of stress when things simply become ambiguous—that is, when things cannot be defined as clearly *either* This *or* That, but rather, when they seem to be *both* This *and* That. In other cases, the dissonance of the world becomes stressful

50. Frenkl-Brunswick, Else. "Intolerance of ambiguity as an emotional and perceptual personality variable." *Journal of Personality*, 18, no. 1 (1949), 108–143.

51. Festinger, L. *A Theory of Cognitive Dissonance*. Palo Alto, CA: Stanford University Press, 1957.

52. Nickerson, Raymond S. "Confirmation bias: A ubiquitous phenomenon in many guises" *Review of General Psychology* 2, no. 2 (June 1998), 175–220.

when our *inner* experience becomes too ambiguous—when we feel two ways about something, as when we feel both compassion and terror in the face of a deadly pandemic.

When life surpasses our tolerance for dissonance and ambiguity, we do not seek resolution by continuing to gather more and more data until a resolution emerges by itself. Instead, we gather information *selectively*, and then we edit that information (sometimes drastically), until it produces a coherent picture that we find acceptable. Some of us even concoct a new reality to achieve a coherent world view. In other words, some of us resort to just making shit up in order to confirm our chosen views. And then we defend what we have concocted as if it were as real as rocks. Satanic pizza parlors. Nano-trackers in our vaccines. Jewish space lasers.

Of course, all of us must edit our data to *some* degree, simply because there is too much information in the world for anyone to compose a completely accurate picture of anything. But *some* folks select and edit their data so profoundly, usually to support some ironclad belief system, that their views of the world eventually bear no detectable resemblance to a commonly shared truth, or what psychologists call "consensual reality."[53] In other words, they construct and live by a version of the world that is fundamentally different from what the vast majority of people would agree is real.

This is how members of the Flat Earth Society can persist in adhering to beliefs that most of us find ludicrous.[54] The same applies to groups who embrace doomsday prophecies that fail to materialize. It also applies to conspiracy cults who treat as fact a variety of long-standing urban myths (satanic cults, child sacrificers, Jewish cabals, etc.) These belief systems always require an us-vs.-them, good-vs.-evil, black-vs.-white lens that simplifies our impossibly complex world. In other words, they are based on a set of simple heuristics that explain everything in theory...and nothing in fact. Tragically, no matter how far-fetched such a belief system may seem to most of us, once it is embraced by emotionally-invested humans, those people will sample only the evidence that confirms their chosen beliefs and they will reject all disconfirming evidence, pursuing "proof" of their bias and

53. Berger, Peter L. and Thomas Luckmann. *The Social Construction of Reality: A Treatise in the Sociology of Knowledge*. Garden City, NY: Anchor Books, 1966.

54. And I do not choose this example randomly, nor should we consider Flat Earthers to be harmless cranks. The pharmacist in Wisconsin who destroyed 500 doses of the Covid-19 vaccine is a devout believer that the Earth is flat…and that the sky is a government-installed shield designed to prevent people from seeing God. See: Salcedo, Andrea. "Wisconsin pharmacist who destroyed more than 500 vaccine doses believes Earth is flat, FBI says." *Washington Post,* February 1, 2021. https://www.washingtonpost.com/nation/2021/02/01/wisconsin-pharmacist-vaccine-flatearth/

constantly re-weaving their cognitive consistency around the world view they have chosen.

What determines the belief system that a given person embraces? The reasons that someone is drawn to any world view, logical or lunatic, have mostly to do with their emotional needs…a topic too complicated to address in this book. But what we *can* address in this book is the way in which people cling to unhelpful stress responses. This usually has much to do with minimizing ambiguity and dissonance, as well as exercising a "confirmation bias" in the way they sample their perceptions of our bewildering world, *especially* under stress.

So let's start with a look at the unhelpful stress responses, giving specific attention to how people have relied on them during pandemics:

Stress responses with commonly unhelpful effects

DENIAL

I could deny it if I liked.
*I could deny **anything** if I liked.*
– Oscar Wilde

The stress response that tempts us all upon the arrival of bad news—especially *really* bad news—is ***denial***. In *denial*, we respond to the stressor by adamantly ignoring or denying its existence. *Denial* can range from asserting that a pandemic disease is "just the flu," or "a liberal hoax," or "too far away to hurt us," all the way to the tragic events reported from South Dakota hospitals in 2020, where devoted constituents of the former president Trump were actively dying of Covid-19 while insisting that it "couldn't be Covid, it has to be the flu, or maybe lung cancer" because Trump had said that the coronavirus wasn't a threat.[55]

The primary (and perhaps only) advantage of *denial* is that it completely removes the source of stress from the consciousness of the person. If there is nothing stressful in our existence, then there is nothing to be stressed about—no plague (Justinian in 547 and the Catholic church in 1347), no

55. Villegas, Paulina. "South Dakota nurse says many patients deny the coronavirus exists—right up until death." *Washington Post*, November 16, 2020. https://www.washingtonpost.com/health/2020/11/16/south-dakota-nurse-coronavirus-deniers/

flu (the governments at war in 1918), no deadly Covid-19 in modern South Dakota. *Denial* offers complete comfort. But that comforting delusion is usually purchased at a very high price...sometimes the highest price, if the stressor being denied is actually a deadly menace.

REGRESSION

Let me not pray to be sheltered from dangers,
but to be fearless in facing them.
– Rabindranath Tagore, ***Fruit Gathering 79***

Closely related to denial is the stress response of ***regression***, in which we react to the stressor by adopting a younger mode of thinking, feeling, or behaving. In other words, we *regress* to a time in our lives before the stressor arrived. *Regression* can convince us that we are safe from the ugly consequences that are looming in the present moment, and we can behave with abandon, as we did when we were children (if we actually *could* behave with abandon when we were children).

One of the more famous historical accounts of *regression* in response to pandemic disease is *The Decameron*, a novel written by Giovanni Boccaccio in 1348, during the height of the Black Death in Italy.[56] In *The Decameron*, seven young women and three young men flee to a villa outside Florence to escape the plague. They spend weeks partying and telling stories of love, lust, conquest, and tragedy, as they are sheltered and pampered by the staff of the villa. *The Decameron* is esteemed as a crucial mirror on the culture of its era, but it also reveals the timeless urge among some people to escape into childlike fantasy when faced with pandemic stress.

Regression does not entirely deny the stressor, but it does create the illusion that one is somehow protected from its dangers, as privileged children are protected from myriad dangers by their childhood caregivers. At the risk of inciting the ire of some readers, it could be said that retreats into religiosity or other devotions to a larger power are examples of regression. Examples would be "I don't need to shelter at home because Jesus will protect me" or "I don't need to wear a mask because President Trump is taking care of the problem" or "I don't need a Covid vaccine because I'm a vegan meditator."

56. Boccaccio, Giovanni. *The Decameron.* Translated and edited by Wayne Rebhorn. New York: W.W. Norton & Co, 1353/2013.

Another example of *regression* is the decision to party with impunity on the beaches of Florida or in the bars of Texas, rebuffing the warnings of public health officials with assertions of one's youthful immunity.

And in case you are wondering about the cultural factors that might correlate with *regression*, there is certainly a valid argument that *regression* is a primary contributor to what has been labeled as "American exceptionalism." This refers to the tendency for many Americans to behave as if we are somehow exempt from the same laws of nature and the same rules of conduct that apply to other peoples (meaning peoples whom we perceive to be "lesser" in resources, privileges, or social status). Exceptionalism has a long and nefarious tradition in human history, stemming from a variety of causes. But for our purposes, the current display of American exceptionalism during the coronavirus pandemic could be interpreted as a kind of adolescent regression into a mindset where one is entitled to flaunt the Covid-prevention guidelines and vaccination advisories because one is somehow immune to a contagion that only affects those less "enlightened" than oneself. (Oh, as if.)

FANTASY AND MAGICAL THINKING

There are two ways to be fooled. One is to believe what isn't true; the other is to refuse to believe what ***is*** *true.*
– Soren Kierkegaard

Another version of acknowledging the stressor while minimizing its danger is to create, endorse, and enact ***fantasy*** versions of the stressful situation, versions that one finds more desirable. This usually means that one's fantasized stressor will bear only the fuzziest resemblance to the actual stressor, and therefore one's response to the actual stressor will be ineffective—sometimes merely useless, but sometimes literally lethal.

Magical thinking gives us the impression that we *are* confronting the stressor and doing something decisive in response to it. The problem with this response is that 1) we usually fantasize the actual stressor as much less dangerous than it actually is, or 2) if our fantasized stressor is just as dangerous as the actual stressor, we make it magically susceptible to the magically powerful countermeasures that we have also fantasized.

During the Black Death, for example, physicians prescribed the carrying of flower bouquets and a blend of herbs to repel the contagion. This is the source of the leading lines in the rhyme, "Ring around the rosy, a pocket full of posies," which alluded to the initial redness of the plague buboes and the flowers to be gathered as prevention of worsening disease. The aromatic flowers did no harm, but they also did nothing to diminish the plague's lethal fire. ("Ashes! Ashes! We all fall *down!*")

Equally quixotic were the masks (also filled with flowers and herbs) that the medieval plague doctors wore to prevent contagion. We can imagine that these masks were quite sobering to the doctors' patients, but they were utterly useless against infection, especially because they had two holes punched in the nose piece that allowed for ventilation…and contagion.

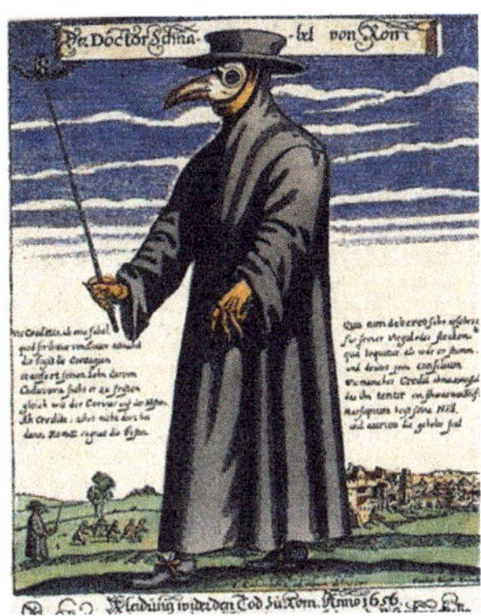

Medieval plague doctor (Wikimedia)

We have seen a wide variety of *magical thinking* responses to the stressor of Covid-19. America's former president Trump spent months imagining the virus to be "just a flu" that would "go away soon." To combat this "flu," Trump proposed a variety of magical remedies, including the irrelevant medicine hydroxycholorquine and the internal administration of household bleach. Trump took hydroxychloroquine himself, to no apparent effect, but some of his supporters followed his second suggestion and ingested bleach, to immediately lethal effect.[57] Other people, those of more progressive beliefs, have endorsed rigorous organic diets, exotic supplements, spiritual exercise, and complementary medical practices as effective replacements for vaccination. All qualify as magical thinking.[58]

DISPLACEMENT

It's too easy to criticize a man when he's out of favor,
and to make him shoulder the blame for
everybody else's mistakes.
– Leo Tolstoy

57. Reimann, Nicholas. "Some Americans Are Tragically Still Drinking Bleach As A Coronavirus 'Cure.'" *Forbes*, Aug 24, 2020. https://www.forbes.com/sites/nicholasreimann/2020/08/24/some-americans-are-tragically-still-drinking-bleach-as-a-coronavirus-cure/?sh=1af5c84c6748

58. Astor, Maggie. "Vocal Anti-vaccine chiropractors split the profession." *New York Times*, July 14 2021. https://www.nytimes.com/2021/07/14/health/anti-covid-vaxxers.html

One of the stress responses that has truly dangerous consequences during pandemics is ***displacement.*** We are displacing our stress when we aim our distressed feelings at a substitute target, rather than the actual source of our stress.

The most common and destructive form of *displacement* during pandemics is the act of *scapegoating*—blaming others for the firestorm of disease and death, even though the others had nothing to do with it. The earliest reference to scapegoating comes from the Bible's book of Leviticus, which describes the Jewish custom of attaching to a goat's hair a variety of tokens that denote one's sins from the past year. The goat is then staked out to die in the wilderness on Yom Kippur (the Day of Atonement), taking the community's sins with him into death and leaving the community cleansed of sin.

Of course, in the ancient Jewish ritual, the members of the community *knew* that the sins borne by the scapegoat were originally *theirs,* and they also knew the goat was doing holy service by dying in order to cleanse them for the coming year.[59] Tragically, in the case of *psychological* scapegoating, the *displacement* onto the scapegoat of blame and related emotions (terror, shame, grief) is entirely *un*conscious, and the scapegoated targets are almost always *human.* The consequence is that those who scapegoat others believe that their targets *deserve* the blame being projected upon them, and they should be punished accordingly.

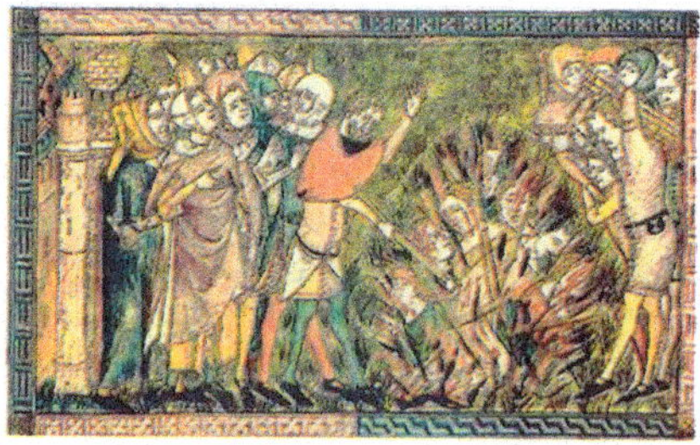
Jewish massacre in Flanders, 1349 CE (Wikimedia)

During the Black Death, for example, tens of thousands of Jews were slaughtered throughout Europe in a frenzy of stress *displacement* and scapegoating. Many Jewish communities—accused of poisoning the city wells, or intentionally infecting others, or killing and drinking the blood of non-Jewish children—were wiped out during the Black Death pandemic. Indeed, many Jews under threat of these horrific massacres committed suicide in order to avoid the attempts of non-Jews to "cleanse" the community by slaughtering Jews by the most heinous means possible. Terror is a searing emotion, but projected terror is utterly incinerating.

59. And yes, this ritual prefigures the Christian role of Jesus, who undergoes death to bear the sins of those who embrace the Christ story, thereby cleansing them of sin so that they can ascend to Heaven.

In the American coronavirus pandemic, we have seen displacement manifested in a variety of ways regarding the contagion of Covid-19. The virus's origins in China have led to some shameful demonstrations of abusive behavior toward Asian Americans.[60] Even former president Trump was fond of scapegoating the people of China for the virus's very existence, referring to it often as "the Chinese virus" and "kung flu." Clearly, human progress in microbiology has not ensured that the regressive stress responses of some people, even those in authority, will keep pace with our species' scientific advances.

PROJECTION

We do not see things as they are. We see things as ***we*** *are.*

– Rabbi Shemuel ben Nachmani (3rd c. CE) [61]

The source of our stress is not the only thing that we tend to avoid. Perhaps even more aversive for some people are the feelings that stress ignites inside us. If we prefer to avoid the feelings of stress, and if we are not familiar with how emotions actually work, then we can fall into the camp of people who use ***projection*** in an attempt to offload their unwanted feelings onto other people. The illusion (usually unconscious) is that one can transfer a load of emotion onto someone else as simply as transferring a backpack of books. Or a bag of boulders. This generally happens in one of two ways...

In the first form of *projection*, we identify someone else who is already displaying feelings that are similar to the feelings we don't want to sense in ourselves. Stressors usually incite feelings of fear (as well as sadness, shame, and surprise), so we usually seek out people who act as if they are experiencing those feelings. Then we point to them and say, "*Those* are the frightened (ashamed, sad, shocked) people. But not *me! I* am doing just fine, thanks. This silly virus can't scare *me!* It's probably just a hoax that has all those spineless snowflakes cowering in their houses

60. Ruiz, Neil, G., Juliana M. Horowitz, and Christine Tamir. "Many black and Asian Americans say they have experienced discrimination amid the COVID-19 outbreak." *PEW Research Center Social & Demographic Trends,* July 1, 2020. https://www.pewresearch.org/social-trends/2020/07/01/many-black-and-asian-americans-say-they-have-experienced-discrimination-amid-the-covid-19-outbreak/

61. *Babylonian Talmud: Tractate Berakoth, Folio 55b.* Translated into English by Maurice Simon, Under the editorship of Rabbi Dr. Isidore Epstein. (Online at halakhah.com – accessed March 8, 2008.)

and covering their faces with masks. But *I'm* not afraid of it! Coronavirus can't hurt *me!* It probably can't hurt them, either. They're just cowards!"

In the second form of *projection*, we take the more dastardly step of *causing* someone else to feel and display our unwanted feelings. For example, we might well be terrified by the deadly virus that is killing the people we love, and we might well be grieving the loss of those people, and we might well be feeling shame about our sense of powerlessness in the face of all of this death and loss. But if we cannot admit or tolerate the fear and grief and shame that we sense under our fearless self-image, then we might do everything we can to *ignite* fear and grief and shame in other people—innocent people—so that we can experience those feelings vicariously. And this simultaneously prevents the projected feelings from tarnishing our sterling self-image. Pretty slick, eh?

This, for example, is one explanation for the intimidation and violence that the anti-mask groups have perpetrated on people who have complied with the protective advisories for minimizing Covid contagion. Challenging the mask-wearing rules in public places produces displays of fear and even terror among the mask-wearers, displays of fear that the anti-maskers appear to find very satisfying. This makes sense because 1) the tactic allows the anti-maskers to experience their fear vicariously through the frightened mask-wearers, and 2) it proves to anti-maskers that *they* are not the frightened ones, like the mask-wearers are. Done and done.

Or it *would* be done...except for the fact that coronavirus doesn't care about projected emotions. Coronavirus only cares about ACE2 receptors, remember? Locate and replicate, replicate, replicate. Thus, the comfort of projected emotion is a very cold kind of comfort when one is facing micro-invaders. For pandemic diseases, "done and done" simply translates into "locate and replicate"—a goal that's much easier for viruses and bacteria to achieve when those pesky masks aren't getting in the way.

So these five responses—*denial, regression, magical thinking, displacement,* and *projection*—are the stress responses whose effects are generally *unhelpful*. Certainly, they are unhelpful to those who employ them. And they can also be unhelpful, even devastating, to the hapless bystanders who are drafted as props and scene partners.

Now let's look at a couple of stress responses that can produce, somewhat randomly, outcomes that are either negative, positive, or simply unremarkable.

Stress responses with unpredictable effects

REPRESSION AND REACTION FORMATION

It is the power of the mind to be unconquerable.
– **Lucius Seneca**, *Stoic Philosophy*

If the emotions that we experience in response to a stressor are deeply uncomfortable, or if they begin to threaten our very sense of self, we may deploy ***repression.*** In this response pattern, we wall off our stress-induced emotions so that they seem not to exist. It is like buckling a suit of emotional armor over one's authentic emotions in an attempt to avoid their distractions or distresses. In *repression*, the emotion that is buckled on over the stress-induced emotion is something like indifference or implacability. People who maintain an "I am a rock" position in the face of impending danger would fall into this category.

Repression can also be manifested as a ***reaction formation***, in which we react in exactly the *opposite* way from what we are naturally feeling. So in a *reaction formation*, the person who is terrified by Covid would act utterly fearless about Covid contagion. This is similar to what happens in the *projection* example above, except that the fearful people who engage in *projection* are not *behaving* fearlessly. They are simply seeking, creating, and then taking comfort in the projected fear they perceive in others. People in *reaction formation* will *behave* fearlessly, regardless of who is around them and how those people are behaving.

Thus, in both *repression* and *reaction formation*, there is no requirement for an innocent bystander who must carry unwanted feelings for the stressed person. Instead, the stressed person has the ability to shield themselves from the true feeling they want to avoid, either by buckling on an armor of no feeling, or else the opposite feeling. If they are afraid, they buckle on a complete lack of emotion, or perhaps a mask of brazen courage, and then they march forward into the fray.

The outcomes of the *repression* and *reaction formation* stress responses vary widely, depending on the circumstances, the emotions, and the persons in which they occur. In the case of deadly pandemics, there are some people, some very heroic people, who buckle on bulletproof calm or bold courage to cover the terror and despair that they naturally feel in the face of overwhelming sickness and death. Then they march forth to save as many people as they possibly can. In the coronavirus pandemic, this would comprise a large percentage of the health care providers and first responders who are placing their lives in jeopardy in order to save the lives of others. During the Black Death, the physician Guy de Chauliac did exactly the same thing, as did many of his peers in medical practice, along with the best of the medieval priests and nuns who tended to the needs of their plague-infected flocks.

The cost of this heroic stress response is that the emotional bill eventually comes due. This is part of what we see in the syndrome we call *post-traumatic stress disorder* (PTSD). The armor of impassivity or courage dissipates after the stressor subsides, allowing the emotional tide to roll in. After the danger has passed, the person is flooded by delayed feelings of terror, grief, shock, and shame (shame often arriving in the form of "survivor's guilt"). These feelings can create serious problems in that person's life, as we have seen in war veterans who suffer from PTSD. However, excellent methods for healing PSTD do exist, so if the post-traumatized person is still alive to feel these postponed emotions, and if the lives of others have been preserved in the process, then *repression* and *reaction formation* can be worth the cost entailed.

Unfortunately, it is also the case that armor buckled over stress feelings can be quite harmful, both for the person wearing the armor and for those nearby. For example, there are people who develop a *reaction formation* by armoring themselves with courage to cover their terror, but who later express that "courage" in acts of tyranny and terrorism. Similarly, those who *repress* their stress-induced feelings and display an impervious lack of reaction—to their own needs or the needs of others—can become dispassionate to the point of lethality.

For all those who respond to stress with *repression* or *reaction formation*, the returning tide of PTSD waits in the moment when stress subsides and leaves room for the original feelings to proceed. Both the "rock" people and the "dauntless" people will be flooded with the emotions they thought they had avoided, emotions that become a challenge to them and/or those near to them. You cannot outrun Mother Nature.

IDENTIFICATION

*Imitation is **not** the sincerest form of flattery.*
*Imitation is the sincerest form of **learning**.*
– George Bernard Shaw

There are times when we respond to a stressor with ***identification***, which is when we adopt the behavior of someone else whom we perceive to be coping successfully with the stress. The challenge with this response is that *identification* will only be as helpful as the stress response of our selected model.

If, for example, we identify with people who react to a stressor with denial of the danger, or with scapegoating of blame (displacement), or with magical thinking, or with projection of their powerless feelings onto despised targets, then we are probably going to experience an outcome of greater sickness and death.

This is, in fact, exactly what happened during the Black Death, when the Roman Catholic Church and local political leaders first denied the danger of the contagion and later responded to the devastation by blaming "the Jewish vermin," exhorting their followers to kill Jews as a means of combatting the plague pandemic. These tactics didn't work in the 14th century, just as making fun of the "kung flu," scapegoating Asians, and eventually endorsing a variety of magical remedies (hydroxychloroquine, ultraviolet light, and household bleach) have only deepened the devastation of coronavirus in America. If we pick the wrong model for our stress response *identification*, we pay a very high price.

If, on the other hand, we identify with people who are responding to a lethal pandemic logically and soberly, with strategies that are informed by good research and rational public health advisors, we are likely to achieve a much more positive outcome.

The greatest challenge with selecting a calm-and-sober model in the face of a lethal pathogen is that the outcome of most calm-and-sober measures is, by definition, a non-event. No dramatic change in our lives. No tidal wave of contagion. No overflowing hospitals and refrigeration trucks full of bodies. No death counts and caseloads in the millions. Calm sobriety is a noble and effective model, but it doesn't grab our attention. It doesn't look as forceful, nor (dare I say it?) as manly in the heat of a pandemic battle. And this makes *identification* a less popular stress response when the stressor is as frightening as a pandemic invader.

At this point, you may be wondering how it is that human beings have ever managed to respond to pandemic stressors with *any* productive outcome. Fortunately, the same ancient forces that installed all of the unhelpful and unpredictable stress responses into our genetic circuits also handed us a few stress responses that were usually beneficial. Nature's sense of humor may be dark, but it is not universally dismal.

Stress responses with generally helpful effects

RATIONAL ANALYSIS

Nothing in life is to be feared; it is only to be understood.
Now is the time to understand more,
so that we may fear less.
– Marie Curie

If there has been one priceless gift of the scientific method, it has been to liberate our ideas about Nature from the chokehold of "confabulation." Confabulation broadly refers to what happens when we really don't know the facts about a complex question, so we just pull an explanation off the ceiling.[62] Sometimes we confabulate consciously in an attempt to gain prestige, or muster confidence, or just preserve our sanity. But sometimes we confabulate without realizing that we are retreating into fiction because we have truly lost our grip on the facts. Brain injuries can do this to us, but so can ignorance and fear.

Rational analysis has afforded humankind a variety of means by which to free ourselves from the pseudo-shelter of our confabulated explanations. By using the skills of 1) careful observation, 2) precise measurement, 3) meticulous record-keeping, 4) mathematical analysis of our records, and 5) conclusions based on logic, we have harvested the rich bounty of modern science—engineering, electronics, and yes, medicine. We now take these treasures for granted, forgetting that most of their gifts have come to us in the last 200 years…a mere blink in the eye of human history.

But just because we have these rational treasures *at* hand, that doesn't mean we always have them *in* hand, especially when a lethal stressor is

62. Confabulation has also been referred to colloquially as "pulling explanations out of one's ass." Or even more colloquially as "making shit up."

terrifying us. As you can imagine, it is very hard for us to maintain a firm grip on the hard facts and a steady hand on the tiller of reason when we are faced with an extreme stressor like a lethal pandemic. We need a hefty dose of the skills we met earlier—*repression* and *positive identification*—both of which allow us to replace our panicky feelings with resolute tenacity and deploy some *rational analysis* to solving the problem.

The medieval doctor Guy de Chauliac appears to have summoned this blend of abilities during the Black Death when he devised his multi-faceted means of combatting plague contagion (as well as a variety of treatments for other maladies). The scientists who have developed, with breathtaking speed, the mRNA vaccines against the coronavirus have summoned a similar set of emotional and intellectual skills.

The enemies of *rational analysis* are mostly our impulsive flares of emotional reactivity. If humankind has one shining advantage (especially because we are so physically vulnerable and easily distractable, as compared to a resilient and monomaniacal virus), it is our capacity for productive reason harnessed to problem-solving determination. Our challenge is to gentle our more primitive urges to bolt, hide, blame, rage, and deny so that our steadier capacities for *rational analysis* can get to work and save our lives.

ANTICIPATION AND PREPARATION

Fortune favors the prepared.
– **Louis Pasteur**

It almost seems too obvious to say that ***anticipation and preparation*** are generally among the most productive responses to stressful events. And yet, some people display a shockingly fierce resistance to the use of these stress responses.

In the realm of deadly pandemic disease, let's consider for a moment the resistance that many people display regarding the most literal and effective form of *anticipation and preparation* once the disease has been scientifically examined and countermeasures have been developed. I'm talking about vaccination, but we could also include the prevention tactics of social distancing, quarantine, and general hygiene.

A safe vaccination for smallpox has been available since the 17th century, and available for most other pandemic diseases for the past 75 years. Effective contagion prevention methods such as quarantine have been available for centuries. Nonetheless, during the coronavirus pandemic in America, some people have displayed a ferocious refusal to engage in any means of *anticipatory preparation.*

The opposition by many Americans to adopt these preventative measures has been a major contributor to the fact that *America, which many believed to have the finest health system and most educated population in the world, has suffered some of the worst Covid statistics on the planet.* This contrast is depicted in the chart below, which compares Covid cases in all world regions by the end of November 2020. The comparison that is most relevant to the issue of *anticipatory preparedness* is the contrast between the statistics for Europe and North America, shown in teal and magenta and fueled in North America primarily by the American case counts, as compared to the statistics for the African continent…shown by the purple line that is well below every other continent except the island "continent" of Oceania.

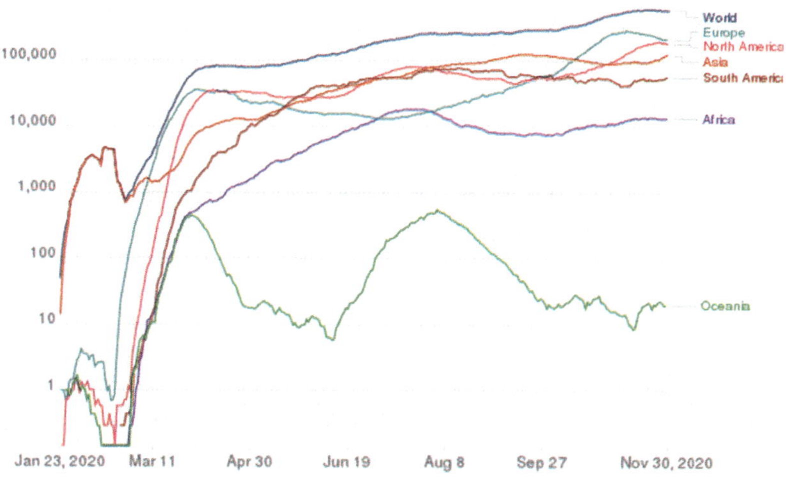

2020 Covid-19 cases by continent (*Our World in Data*). (Wikimedia)

By many measures, the social resources of the North American continent exceed those of the African continent. But as we now know, material wealth does not compensate for a poverty of wisdom and pragmatism. Most analysts now agree that Africa is receiving the benefit of the following factors in its fight against Covid:[63]

63. Barker, Aryn. "Why Africa's COVID-19 Outbreak Hasn't Been as Bad as Everyone Feared." *Time*, December 30, 2020. https://time.com/5919241/africa-covid-19-outbreak/

1. A well-developed public health system that must proactively compensate for the continent's lack of more advanced medical care,
2. A younger population that is more resistant to infection,
3. A long and diverse experience with deadly pandemics, such as Ebola virus, and therefore,
4. *A highly sensitive and well-developed response of anticipation and preventative preparation, both among the African health care workers and among the African peoples in general.*

In other words, if we don't count South Africa, the African peoples have greatly surpassed Americans in their ability to exercise the stress response of *anticipatory preparation.* Partly as a result of that response, their Covid statistics have been among the best in the world...while the American statistics are the worst. Strike a match on *that.*

HUMOR

Two things are infinite: the universe and human stupidity.
And I'm not sure about the universe.
– **Albert Einstein**[64]

I know it may be hard to believe, but another potent weapon that we have when responding to any stressor, and especially stressors of the microscopically contagious variety, is our capacity for *humor*. In an act of supreme scholastic courage, the marketing and psychology professor Peter McGraw has concisely defined humor as what occurs when something entails a balanced amount of threat and safety. Things cease to be funny, McGraw asserts, when they become either too threatening or too benign.[65] This simple definition of a phenomenon as complex as humor seems a bit glib at first chuckle, but upon reflection, one has to admit that McGraw has a point.

The reason that humor can be such a helpful stress response is because it places the stressor in a larger perspective, enabling us amused humans to regain some sense that there is a bigger context from which to view and solve the frightening problem. In other words, humor makes the threatening stressor appear a little less terrifying, thus allowing us to preserve our wits,

64. Cited in Perls, Fritz. *In and Out the Garbage Pail.* Zurich: Gestalt Journal Press, 1969.
65. McGraw, A. Peter and Joel Warner. *The Humor Code: A Global Search for What Makes Things Funny.* New York, NY: Simon & Schuster, 2014.

as well as our wit, for the essential task of pandemic problem-solving. (Humor may also ignite our crucial creative capacities in that same task… but more on that later.)

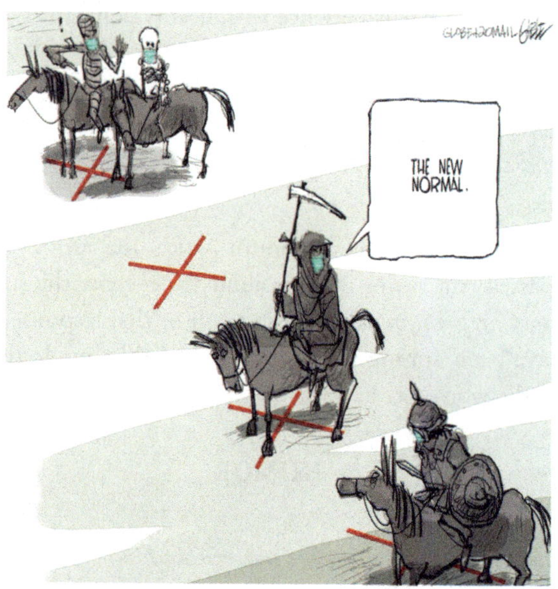

© 2020 Brian Gable, *The Canadian Globe and Mail*

For example, you surely remember the four apocalyptic equestrians from the beginning of this chapter…those dealers of death that we humans have feared for millennia. Shown above are those same four Horsemen, drawn by the brilliant political cartoonist Brian Gable in reference to the coronavirus pandemic. Yes, that would be Pestilence holding the scythe, with War in the lower right and the skeleton of Famine at the top, exasperating Death by violating his social distancing space in an attempt to avoid Pestilence. And all four Horsemen are, of course, wearing the obligatory aqua medical masks. No one is excluded from observing pandemic protocols, not even the mounted Destroyers.[66]

Gable produced this cartoon during the first spasm of terrorized pandemic sheltering, when no one knew what degree of viral devastation was headed our way. To be able to laugh at ourselves in the midst of this lethally grim situation was a balm for our souls and a reprieve for our overheated immune systems. (Because laughter is also excellent immune support. But you knew that already, right?)

66. © 2020 by Brian Gable, *The Canadian Globe and Mail.* Originally published May 14, 2020. Reprinted by permission of The Canadian Press Enterprises, Inc.

SUBLIMATION

A rock pile ceases to be a rock pile the moment a single man contemplates it, bearing within him the image of a cathedral.

– Antoine de Saint-Exupery[67]

Given all of the regrettable (albeit understandable) stress responses that human beings display when we're faced with really bad news, it is something of a miracle that any of us manage to summon forth the response that transcends even the benign responses of rationality, preparation, and wit. In the midst of a terrified throng that is afflicted by denial, scapegoating, fantastic delusions, and outright terror, a few intrepid souls always emerge and arrange their wits into some semblance of productive sanity. These are the people who, when faced with a pile of rocks, or boulders, or lava bombs, resist the urge to join the panicking mob. Instead, they somehow manage to perceive, and even produce, a transcendent cathedral.

This is the stress response that is called ***sublimation***, derived from the word "sublime"—to be uplifting, inspiring, transcendent. All pandemics inundate us with sickness, suffering, terror, and death. They are the inevitable curses of pestilential contagion. The ability to rise above that miasma of affliction and derive a transcendent vision is a precious gift—a gift to oneself and a gift to those with whom one shares the vision. And the gift is even more precious when one's vision can be transformed into a means of practical relief to those who are afflicted.

Historically, those who have been capable of practical *sublimation* have been the heroic human defenders in the war against pandemic disease. And rest assured that I do *not* include in this noble clan the mob mongers who spew words of false blame, false prophecy, or false reassurance. By contrast, Edward Jenner's refinement of the smallpox vaccine is one example of pandemic heroism. Another is Ignaz Semmelweis, who introduced methods of antiseptic procedure into the contagion swamp of archaic medical practice. Semmelweis's fierce campaign against sepsis has led to the hygienic protocols that are powerful weapons in pandemic prevention.

In the coronavirus pandemic, the microbiologists like Katalin Karikó and Drew Weissman, who have developed with blazing speed the various

67. De Saint-Exupéry, Antoine. *Le Petit Prince*. Paris: Gallimard, 1943.

vaccines we can now deploy against the coronavirus are also members of that sublimating army.[68] So are the public health researchers and advocates, like Dr. Anthony Fauci, who have courageously advocated for the techniques of hygiene, social distancing, contagion tracking, and quarantine—our best allies in the absence of, and in support of, any vaccines against deadly pandemic disease. And so are the scientists who are developing the use of "nanobodies" to neutralize a coronavirus infection after it has happened.[69]

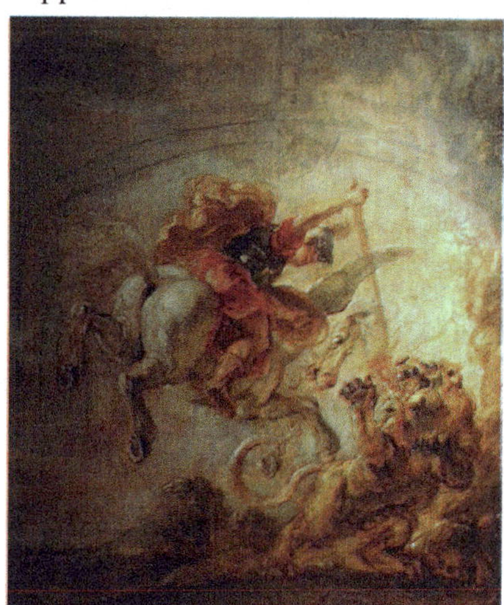

Bellerophon and Pegasus swoop down to kill the Chimera (Rubens, 1635) (Wikimedia)

To grasp the essence of the sublimating pandemic antagonist, let's return to the last chapter, when we met the mythic destroyer Chimera, whose lethal campaign roared unchecked against all countermeasures. All countermeasures, that is, that could not attain an elevated perspective on the deadly beast. But when Bellerophon arrived, mounted on the winged Pegasus, he was able to observe and attack the Chimera from a higher vantage point. He also was able to maintain the presence of mind necessary to aim and plunge a wad of lead into the fire-breathing maw of the ram in the middle of the monster.

This is *sublimation*—the ability to perceive and manifest an effective response to the source of one's stress. The sublimated response could be something as concrete as developing a healthy exercise program when sheltering at home through the pandemic, as innovative as crafting an online format for practicing one's profession, as small (and comforting) as learning to do one's own manicure, or as world-changing as creating an mRNA vaccine against a deadly virus.

Sublimation usually requires some measure of the other helpful stress

68. Goldman, Bruce. "How do the new Covid-19 vaccines work?" *Scope,* December 22, 2020. https://scopeblog.stanford.edu/2020/12/22/how-do-the-new-covid-19-vaccines-work/

69. Piore, Adam. "A UCSF team has engineered a tiny antibody capable of neutralizing the coronavirus." *University of California San Francisco*, February 4, 2021. https://www.universityofcalifornia.edu/news/

responses, including the abilities to contain one's fear, deploy one's reason, and retain one's wits...and wit (remembering that humor grants elevated perspective by reducing the perceived danger of the threat). It is the response in which we meet the stressor factually, courageously, creatively, and in the best of outcomes, successfully. The more we can sublimate, the more successful and satisfied we are likely to be with our outcomes—in our relationships, in our work, in our lives, and in our global pandemics.

♦ ♦ ♦

So here we are...We have met the microscopic invader of this story—the novel coronavirus—and we have met its most famous predecessors in the history of human pandemic diseases.

We have learned something about the antecedents to the current pandemic and the antecedents to the four firestorms of disease that have preceded it in human history, including the ways in which those four pandemic stories bear uncanny resemblances to our own.

We have become acquainted with our microscopic defenders—the infinitesimal but ferocious warriors of the human immune system who launch their full selves against the disease invaders of every pandemic in a valiant effort to save the human body (despite the tragic fact that their heroic campaign often kills us in the process).

And we have learned about the diverse things that are done by the macro-defenders of our story—we human beings who suffer and die by the millions, but who also dare to fight back against the diseases that are slaughtering us.

Now it is time to look at some essential stories from each pandemic... the historical pandemic stories, and also the story of this novel coronavirus pandemic, primarily in America. As we have seen, no one pandemic story is entirely separate from any other, especially when those stories share a common kind of invader, a common set of defenders, and so many common elements of precedent and causation.

So as we recount each pandemic story, as we explore each narrative of essence, we will be living them all. And all these pandemic stories will be telling *us* something, too. Because isn't that how stories work? We think that we are simply telling a few compelling stories. But in fact, they are simultaneously telling *us*...telling us what we yearn to know, telling us what we hope to learn, and telling us what we desperately need to witness, if only we have the courage to see it.

Let us enter the tales...

CHAPTER 5

Four Stories Left for Us by the Victims and Survivors of Pandemics

History is written by the winners.
– Author unknown, ca. 18th century CE

History is not written by the winners.
History is written by the survivors.
– Jay Price, Director of Public History, Wichita State University[70]

History is written by the writers.
– Lance Strate, Professor of Communication and Media Studies, Fordham University[71]

There is no such thing as an accurate account of a historic human event. Life and the people who live it are too subtle and too complex. All we can document about any event, even the simplest event, is the skin on the beast of the story. But the story itself is too rich and paradoxical to be recounted scientifically—not even if you use a fountain of facts or a plethora of pictures. Trying to convey a historic event by using only its facts is like trying to convey a tiger by dissecting it down to its cells. What you have left is just tiger mush, bearing little resemblance to Tiger. Which is what we can imagine William Blake had in mind when he wrote this poem...

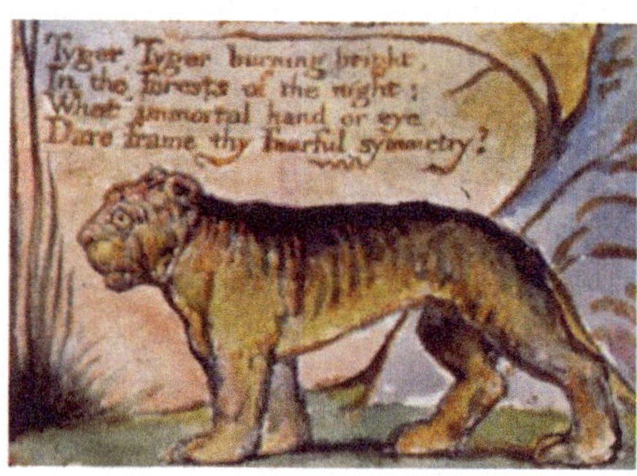

Tyger Tyger burning bright,
In the forests of the night;
What immortal hand or eye,
Dare frame thy fearful symmetry?
"Tyger, Tyger!" William Blake, *Songs of Experience* (1794) (Wikimedia)

A global pandemic is among the largest of historic events...a veritable tiger of an event. This

70. https://www.wichita.edu/about/wsunews/news/2020/08-aug/somos_9.php
71. http://lancestrate.blogspot.com/2010/01/hisotry-is-written-by-writers-not.html

means that pandemics are especially resistant to accurate reporting. Fortunately, most of us aren't seeking a thoroughly accurate account of any historic event, even a global pandemic that has killed millions of our fellow humans. What most of us are seeking is the *story* of the historic event. In other words, we are seeking a narrative of the event that captures its *essence*.

In 1957, the Cuban poet/novelist José Lezama Lima described history as a "shared memory" that eventually becomes a "consensual narrative."[72] According to Lima's compelling proposal, the facts of any historical record are embellished by its narrators with ancient images and cherished storylines, creating a version of the historical truth that is evocative and enduring for the people who retain it, despite the fact that it is *never* a precise record of what actually happened.

William Shakespeare had a superb grasp on this definition of history. Partly because his work had to win the approval of the reigning English monarch, but also because he cherished a good story, Shakespeare wrote versions of historical events that have (to the exasperation of many historians) surpassed and outlived the facts of the actual events—events to which his stories bore only passing resemblance.

To this day, for example, there remains a heated debate about whether or not King Richard III was the demonic psychopath who ordered the Tower of London murder of those two precious princes (his nephews, to be precise).[73] [74]

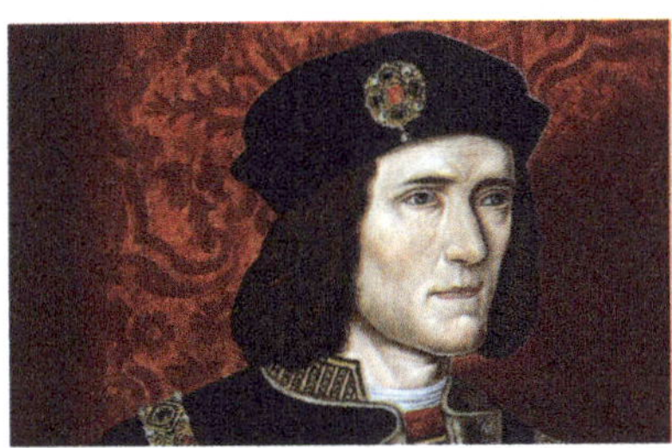

King Richard III, Artist unknown (1510-1540) (Wikimedia)

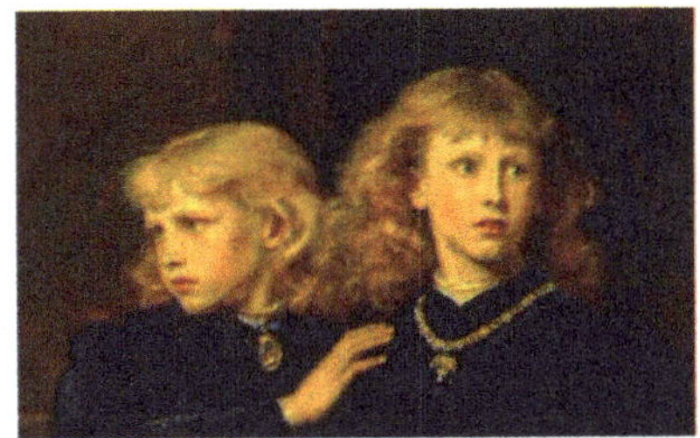

The Princes in the Tower, John Millais (1878) (Wikimedia)

72. Lezama Lima, José. *La expresión americana*. Irlemar Chiampi: México, Fondo de Cultura Económica, 1957/2001.

73. Thornton, Tim. "More on a Murder: The Deaths of the 'Princes in the Tower' and Historiographical Implications for the Regimes of Henry VII and Henry VIII." *Journal of the Historical Association,* December 28, 2020. New York: Wiley & Sons Online. https://onlinelibrary.wiley.com/doi/full/10.1111/1468-229X.13100

74. Tey, Josephine. *The Daughter of Time.* London: Peter Davies, 1951.

Based on the most current research, it appears that Richard was not a satanic monster.[75] But the "consensual narrative" that endures about Richard is the murderous tale that Shakespeare composed for Queen Elizabeth I—the queen who was Shakespeare's patron and who was also descended from the branch of the feuding royal family that was *opposed* to Richard's. Elizabeth's side of the family were the survivors and the winners, so it was on behalf of their lineage and reputation that Shakespeare was hired to write his history plays.

So it was that a heart-wrenching version of a historic event was composed by a writer (a *superb* writer, at that) who worked for the people who were both the winners *and* the survivors of the event. Historians are still arguing about what really happened during the reign of Richard III, and it's possible that no one will ever know for sure. The story that prevails in the minds of most people, however, is the searing tale that Shakespeare wrote about a ruthless powermonger who was ready to annihilate anyone, including innocent children, who stood between himself and the crown. And let's be honest; it's hard for mere reality to compete with the rich verse of that bloody saga...

> And thus I clothe my naked villany
> With old odd ends stolen out of holy writ;
> And seem a saint, when most I play the devil.
>
> *The Tragedy of King Richard III*, I.iii

When we turn to the history of pandemics, we see similar distortions in the storytelling. But in the case of pandemic disease, the distortions tend toward minimizing and even obliterating, rather than aggrandizing and myth-making. Pandemic events have rarely been given a central role in historical stories. Perhaps this was because disease and death were much more pervasive during the four historic pandemics I have described. Or perhaps it's because (to invoke Camus) "pestilence isn't a thing made to man's measure."[76] If we follow Lima's theory that history is a "consensual narrative" that is co-created by the people who lived through the event, it may be that those who survived these firestorms of pestilence had no means (and perhaps no desire) to convey their experience with a mere line of words...even a long and tragic line of words.

75. Skidmore, Chris. *Richard III: England's Most Controversial King.* New York: St. Martin's Press, 2018.

76. Camus, Albert. (1947) *The Plague (La Peste)* Vintage, New York, NY. p. 37

Shakespeare himself mentioned plague seldom in his entire canon, and then only briefly, despite the fact that surges of actual plague were closing down the theaters during Shakespeare's life, once for as long as 30 months. Modern historians who write about the Black Death have lamented the scarcity of 14th century accounts about that pandemic, even though we know that it killed half of Europe and perhaps a third of the rest of the world. Similarly, there is only one substantial written document that survives from the plural pandemics of the post-Columbian New World, and no accounts that fully convey the extent of that human catastrophe. Even in modern history, which offers us a wealth of documentation on most subjects, the global disaster that was inflicted by *influenza H1N1* from 1918 to 1920 was *never* explicitly described, nor fully comprehended, until fifty years after it occurred.

So who composes the essential narrative of a pandemic and where do we find those stories?

Certainly, modern historians do their best to offer us the facts pertaining to the historic pandemics. They give us dates and names of the afflicted people of the time (only the famous people, of course, never the anonymous millions who suffered and died). And they give us some evidence about the micro-invader's assault on the human terrain it is conquering—that is, the physical symptoms of disease and death that they have deduced from their research. Historians also chart the invader's geographic march, mapping its campaign of contagion. And they report some of the things that the human defenders did in response to the pathogen's invasion. Historians also like to tell us about their more common subjects of interest—the social and environmental events that were occurring while the microscopic invaders were mowing down the population.

Some of the things that historians tell us end up in what Lima would call the "consensual narrative" of a pandemic. But even those carefully researched facts are fodder for ongoing debate. In the end, the heart of the matter seems to be less about who gives us the most *accurate* history of a pandemic (or any event), and more about who can absorb the ocean of data and distill from it a narrative that conveys the *essence* of the story. Of course, no single consensual narrative can capture the totality of any historic event, especially an event as complex as a global pandemic. Nonetheless, we *can* identify narratives that carry some key portion of a pandemic's essence, narratives that transcend time and locale to convey an elemental truth about that particular inferno of disease. Let's look at four of those narratives.

A Story from the Plague of Justinian

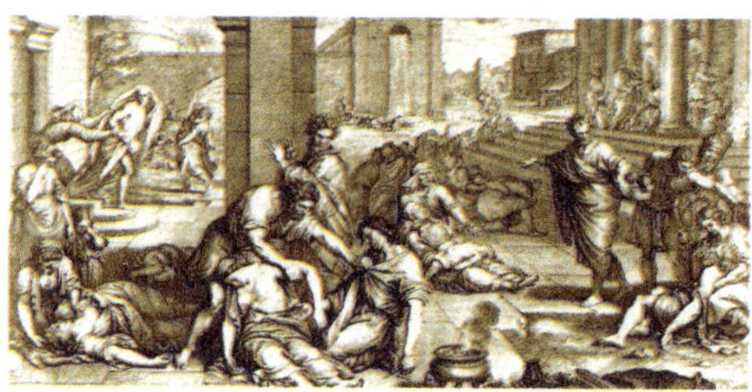

The Plague of Epirus, Pierre Mignard (1612-1695)
(Wikimedia)

As you probably remember from the chapter on how pandemics begin, the Plague of Justinian was the first global pandemic in human history that was explicitly recorded. It was a pandemic of *yersinia pestis* that struck the Mediterranean region in 541 CE and decimated much of the ancient world. It also decimated the vaulting ambitions of Emperor Justinian, whose life goal (and nearly his accomplishment) was to resurrect the Roman Empire. We know that ancient peoples were familiar with outbreaks of pandemic disease long before plague struck down Justinian's empire. The apocalyptic horseman Pestilence shows up in books of the Old Testament that date back to the 5th century BCE, which tells us that the threat of contagion was far older than its biblical debut. For example, as many as 100,000 people died of some disease (not plague, but possibly a viral hemorrhagic fever) in the "Plague of Athens" in 430 BCE. However, the evidence that is left to us about the Plague of Justinian indicates that it was the first pandemic in which we see evidence of the notion that a pestilence could "end the world," or at any rate, that it could end the world as it was known to its current inhabitants.[77]

One major challenge with tracking down any ancient narrative is that the people living in antiquity possessed limited methods by which they could preserve their stories for millennial posterity. We can suppose, therefore, that there were countless songs, stories, poems, and plays that were composed in memory of that 6th century pandemic...the first cataclysmic war between a

77. Specifically, even during the Plague of Athens, it was known that *only* Athenians were dying of the disease that afflicted them. The Spartans, who had laid siege to Athens, fled home and there is no record that the contagion spread to them or any other peoples outside of Africa, from which the disease arrived by ship, according to the historian Thucydides. (*History of the Peloponnesian War* 2.48.1)

disease invader and its human defenders. But nearly all of those memorial creations fell victim to their own ephemeral natures; that is, they survived only as long as they could be performed or recounted, and nothing remains of them for us to explore.[78]

Therefore, we who regard antiquity from this vast temporal distance must cherish and rely upon the sparse stories that were recorded in a durable form. These are the narratives, including those of the Justinian Plague, whose original copies were mostly lost, but not until they had been carefully copied by monastic scribes, those faithful chroniclers who preserved through subsequent centuries the ancient works we do have.

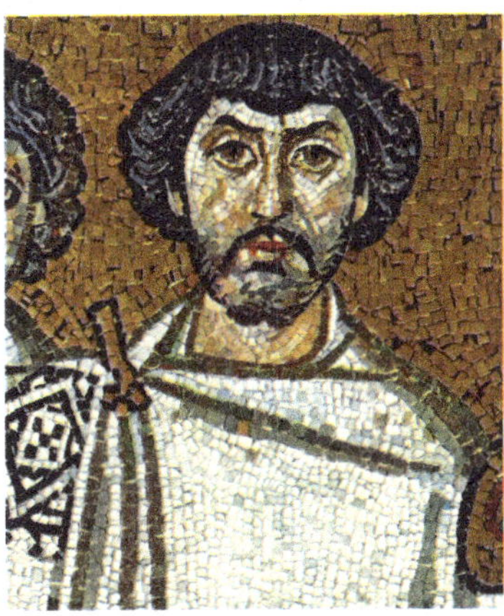

Procopius, from a mosaic in the Church of San Vitale, Ravenna, Italy (547 CE) (Wikimedia)

Our primary narrator about the Justinian pandemic is the Byzantine scholar Procopius of Caesaria, who is commonly considered to be the last major historian of the ancient Western world. Some recent historians have challenged the narrative of Procopius, claiming that certain current evidence, added to his dislike of his imperial boss Justinian, diminishes the credibility of his story.[79] But Procopius's description is uncannily consistent with comparable accounts from pandemics like the Black Death and the 1918 flu. These powerful similarities challenge the critiques of contemporary historians, who are obliged to look through modern lenses when they evaluate ancient experience. In rebuttal to these recent critiques, many scholars feel that it looks like Procopius was recounting what he saw as truthfully as he saw it, adding only the biases of horror and disbelief that would distort the account of any normal person who was witnessing and reporting such hideous things on such a massive scale...for the first time in

78. It is important to remember here that the Greeks assigned their nine Muses—the demi-gods of the ancient arts—only to the arts that were *ephemeral* in antiquity. These were comedy, tragedy, dance, music, love poetry, epic poetry, sacred stories, astronomy/astrology... and *history*. Thus, the Muses gave divine blessing to the creative works that could not live longer than their human embodiment. And because history in antiquity was most often conveyed by oral narration, the ancients considered it primarily an ephemeral creation, along with the related traditions of song, dance, poem, and story.

79. Mordechai, Lee, Merle Eisenberg, Timothy Newfield, Adam Izdebski, Janet Kay, and Hendrik Poinar. "The Justinianic Plague: An inconsequential pandemic?" *Proceedings of the National Academy of Sciences*, December 17, 2019. https://doi.org/10.1073/pnas.1903797116

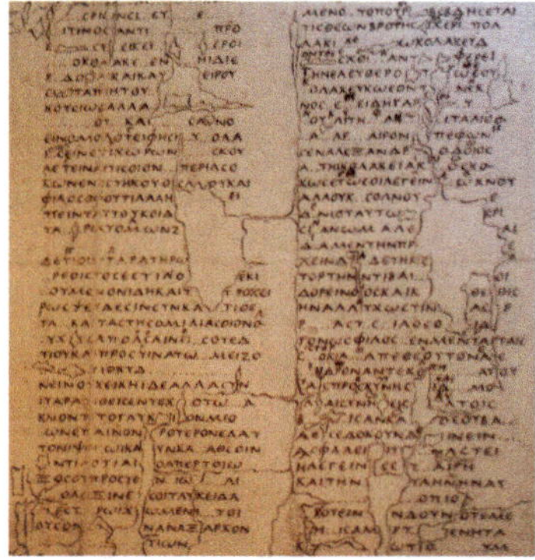

Greek manuscript from 6th century CE, contemporary with Procopius' long-vanished manuscript describing the Justinian Plague (Wikimedia)

recorded history.

Although the following excerpts are lengthy, I want to include these portions of Procopius's account of the Justinian Plague, partly because this is the only concise account of these events, and also because this narrative is tragically compelling and eerily modern, even after 1500 years:

During these times there was a pestilence by which the whole human race came near to being annihilated. Now, in the case of all other scourges sent from heaven, some explanation of a cause might be given by daring men... But for this calamity it is quite impossible either to express in words or to conceive in thought any explanation, except indeed to refer it to God....For it seemed to move by fixed arrangement, and to tarry for a specified time in each country, casting its blight slightingly upon none, but spreading in either direction right out to the ends of the world, as if fearing lest some corner of the earth might escape it...

With the majority it came about that they were seized by the disease without becoming aware of what was coming... They had a sudden fever, some when just roused from sleep, others while walking about, and others while otherwise engaged, without any regard to what they were doing. And the body showed no change from its previous color, nor was it hot as might be expected when attacked by a fever, nor indeed did any inflammation set in, but the fever was of such a languid sort, from its commencement and up till evening, that neither to the sick themselves nor to a physician who touched them would it afford any suspicion of danger.

It was natural, therefore, that not one of those who had contracted the disease expected to die from it. But on the same day in some cases, in others on the following day, and in the rest not many days later, a bubonic swelling developed; and this took place not only in the particular part of the body which is called boubon, *that is, "below the abdomen," but also inside the armpit, and in some cases also beside the ears, and at different points on the thighs. Up to this point, then, everything went in about the same way with all who had taken the disease.*

But from then on very marked differences developed... For there ensued with some a deep coma, with others a violent delirium, and in either case they suffered the characteristic symptoms of the disease. For those who were under the spell of the coma forgot all those who were familiar to them and seemed to lie sleeping constantly. And if anyone cared for them, they would eat without waking... But those who were seized with delirium suffered from insomnia and were victims of a distorted imagination; for they suspected that men were coming upon them to destroy them, and they would become excited and rush off in flight, crying out at the top of their voices.

Death came in some cases immediately, in others after many days. And with some the body broke out with black pustules about as large as a lentil, and these did not survive even one day, but all succumbed immediately. With many also a vomiting of blood ensued without visible cause and straightway brought death.

And at first the deaths were a little more than the normal, then the mortality rose still higher, and afterwards the tale of dead reached five thousand each day, and again it even came to ten thousand and still more than that. In the beginning, each man attended to the burial of the dead of his own house, and these they threw even into the tombs of others, either escaping detection or using violence. But afterwards confusion and disorder everywhere became complete...

When it came about that all the tombs which had existed previously were filled with the dead, then they dug up all the places about the city one after the other, laid the dead there, each one as he could, and departed... They piled them up just as each one happened to fall, and filled practically all the towers with corpses, and then covered them again with their roofs. As a result of this an evil stench pervaded the city and distressed the inhabitants still more, and especially whenever the wind blew fresh from that quarter.

And work of every description ceased, and all the trades were abandoned by the artisans, and all other work as well, such as each had in hand. Indeed, in a city which was simply abounding in all good things, starvation almost absolute was running riot. Certainly, it seemed a difficult and very notable thing to have a sufficiency of bread or of anything else.

Such was the course of the pestilence in the Roman Empire at large as well as in Byzantium. And it fell also upon the land of the Persians and visited all the other barbarians besides.[80]

80. Procopius. *History of the Wars*, Volume 1, Books 1 & 2. Translated by H. B. Dewing. Cambridge, MA: Harvard University Press, 1914.

Whatever Procopius's biases may have been, it is hard to read this passage and dismiss it as the wanton exaggeration of a political pundit. This is the voice of a witness to a pestilential horror that had never been chronicled before...that had, in fact, never before been imagined or experienced to this degree. This is a voice speaking the essence of a ghastly truth.

Of course, the facts of the Justinian Plague were far more complicated, though no less tragic, than what we receive from Procopius in this grim story—a narrative that seizes our hearts from across the span of fifteen centuries. We know we have encountered a narrative of essence when the words of the narrator, so far removed from us, feel immediate and heartbreaking. Fortunately, we have this one man, known to us only from a single mosaic and his anguished words, to remind us that consciousness and compassion have always been available to human beings, even when we have been tempted to retreat blindly into denial, despair, and death. The witnessing of our darkest moments—courageous witnessing with both mind and heart, even if we are powerless to change what we witness—is among the most sublime gifts of our species.

A Story from the Black Death

Eight hundred years after *yersinia pestis* had burned through the population of the known world, it returned again for a second campaign of conquest. Stoked by the forces we learned about in the chapter on how pandemics begin, the plague's second European campaign ignited in Italy, in 1347. Although the worst of its incendiary damage was done in its first five years, subsequent waves of plague swept through Europe for the next 400 years. (Yes, *400 years.*)

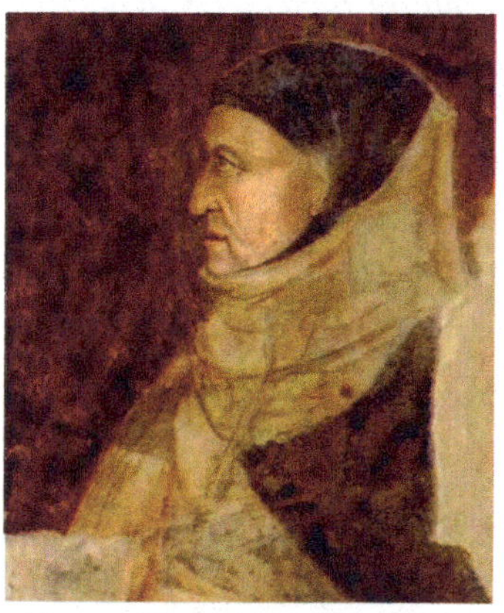

Giovanni Boccaccio (c. 1370) Galleria Uffizi, Florence, Italy (Wikimedia)

A variety of stories have been penned about the Black Death, but the most iconic is found in Giovanni Boccaccio's *The Decameron*, which I mentioned earlier. In *The Decameron,* Boccaccio invites us to a gathering of seven young women and three young men who have fled the plague to a country villa outside of Florence. Most of the book is devoted to the stories that these privileged evacuees compose for their entertainment. But Bocaccio also included in *The Decameron* the most comprehensive report of contemporary experience during the first onslaught of the Black Death. I am not selecting these excerpts as the "consensual narrative" for this pandemic, but they merit inclusion, if only to confirm the validity of Procopius's description, which they echo to a horrifying (though unsurprising) degree.

The violence of this disease was such that the sick communicated it to the healthy who came near them, just as a fire catches anything dry or oily near it. And it even went further. To...touch the clothes or anything else the sick had touched or worn gave the disease to the person touching...

Such terror was struck into the hearts of men and women by this calamity, that brother abandoned brother, and the uncle his nephew, and the sister her brother, and very often the wife her husband. What is even worse and nearly incredible is that fathers and mothers refused to see and tend their children, as if they had not been theirs....

Some thought that moderate living and the avoidance of all superfluity would preserve them from the epidemic... Others thought just the opposite. They thought the sure cure for the plague was to drink and be merry... Many others adopted a course of life midway between the two just described...they did not shut themselves up, but went about, carrying flowers or scented herbs or perfumes in their hands, in the belief that it was an excellent thing to comfort the brain with such odors; for the whole air was infected with the smell of dead bodies, of sick persons and medicines...

It made no difference. Dead bodies filled every corner. Such was the multitude of corpses brought to the churches every day and almost every hour that there was not enough consecrated ground to give them burial... Because the cemeteries were full, they were forced to dig huge trenches where they buried the bodies by hundreds. Here they stowed them away like bales in the hold of a ship and covered them with a little earth, until the whole trench was full. [81]

This is probably the closest we will ever get to a contemporary historical account of the Black Death. However, millions of words in both fiction and nonfiction have been written on the subject since Bocaccio wrote these.[82]

81. Boccaccio, Giovanni. *The Decameron.* Translated by Wayne Rebhorn. New York: W.W. Norton & Co, 1353/2013.

82. My three preferred books about the Black Death are John Kelly's brilliant historical treatment *The Great Mortality: An Intimate History of the Black Death, the Most Devastating Plague of All Time* (San Francisco: HarperCollins, 2005), Barbara Tuchman's comprehensive tour of the 14th century (including the Black Death) *A Distant Mirror: The Calamitous Fourteenth Century* (New York: Alfred A. Knopf, 1978), and Connie Willis' astonishing novel *Doomsday Book* (New York: Bantam, 1992).

Oddly, the Black Death pandemic (or "second plague," as it is officially called by historians) has not been accorded a literary treatment as memorable or majestic as *The Tragedy of King Richard III.* (Once again, it's most regrettable that Shakespeare never wrote a play about a pandemic.) However, we do have one compelling story from the Black Death...remarkably compelling because it was only recorded in a set of accounting books.[83] This story offers such an iconic portrait of its time, and it demands such a personal relationship with its audience, that it could well be considered an example of Lima's "consensual narrative." Let's follow the plague's European pilgrimage to this oddly symbolic tale.

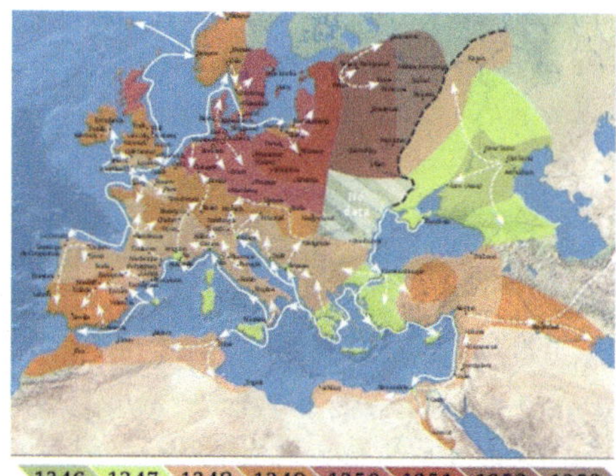

(Wikimedia)

During its second global campaign, *yersinia pestis* made first land in European bodies during 1347 arriving in Sicily on a ship from Constantinople. By the standards of the time, the plague blazed across Europe with lightning speed. But the relatively small populations and limited means of travel in medieval Europe slowed its transmission drastically compared to what we would see today. Covid-19 circled the globe in mere weeks in the 21st century, but in the 14th century, it took several years for the plague to cross Europe. However, one thing that has *not* changed about pandemic contagion since the Middle Ages is that not all sectors of a pandemic world are equally afflicted. For example, it is still unknown why Poland was spared the worst of the Black Death.

Sadly, southeast England was not so lucky. Historians believe that the southeastern portion of England suffered an especially cruel assault during the early years of the plague, possibly because there was an outbreak of a livestock disease (perhaps anthrax) at the same time that the plague was

83. We should not be surprised that a set of accounting records could convey the essence of a historical event. To quote the historian Barbara Tuchman, "Disaster is rarely as pervasive as it seems from recorded accounts. The fact of [a disaster] being on the record makes it appear continuous and ubiquitous, whereas it is more likely to have been sporadic both in time and place." (Ibid. p. xviii). Tuchman paid great attention to accounting records, because she felt that the records of commerce would yield a more comprehensive and accurate picture of contemporary events, especially during "calamitous" periods like the Black Death.

ravaging the land. Privations from an earlier famine and years of war had also created intense social unrest, which resulted in "the Peasants' Revolt of 1381." So, the people were stressed, the animals were stressed, the social order was stressed...and then came the plague. In sum, while every pandemic is horrible, the Black Death in southeastern England was nothing short of hell on Earth.

And here is where our story begins...[84]

About 35 miles southwest of London is the market town of Farnham, which in 1348 was the seat of "the Hundred at Farnham"—one of the richest and most populous estates in southeastern England. The Farnham estate was run by a "reeve," newly employed in his position in 1348. A reeve was like a cross between a steward and a magistrate, and in this case, he was a young man by the name of John Ronewyk.

The facts we have about John himself are few, so we must flesh out his character from the facts we have about Farnham and its management. Happily, these facts are numerous, partly because Farnham's story is contained in its vast bookkeeping records (John was an excellent bookkeeper), and partly because of the plain dumb luck that those bookkeeping records didn't vanish during the subsequent 800 years.

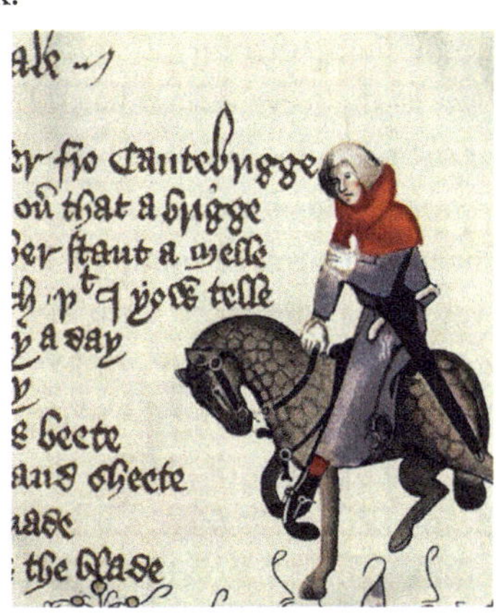

The Reeve, Geoffrey Chaucer, *The Canterbury Tales* (c. 1400 CE) (Wikimedia)

John's record of his Farnham story is literally written on fragile scrolls called "the Winchester Pipe Rolls"—long pieces of parchment that documented in detail the operation of properties like the Hundred at Farnham. From these meticulous records (which John maintained by order of the King), we observe a statistical portrait of life at Farnham during the worst of the Black Death. And those Pipe Roll's

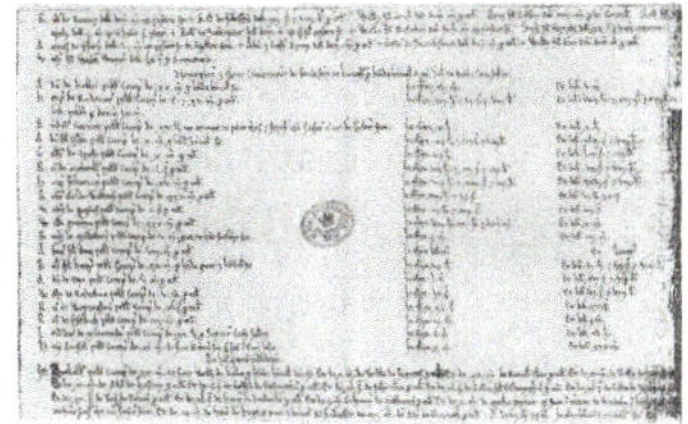

An example of a medieval "pipe roll" --» an accounting record kept by royal order, like the records created by John Ronewyk (Wikimedia)

84. I am greatly indebted to John Kelly's *The Great Mortality* (*op. cit.*) for introducing me to John Ronewyk, and I'm subsequently grateful for the details contained in the historical document by E. Robo, "The Black Death in the Hundred of Farnham" (*The English Historical Review*, Vol. XLIV, Issue CLXXVI, October 1929, pp. 560–572. https://academic.oup.com/ehr/article-abstract/XLIV/CLXXVI/560/489211)

statistics allow us to flesh out with confidence the humanity in the rest of the story.

An estate like Farnham was not just a workplace. It comprised farmland for raising crops, pastureland for raising livestock, buildings to house the work of farming and husbandry, and villages in which the workers lived with their families. Farnham was, in fact, the place in which these workers lived out their entire lives. No vacations. No "trips to town." No evenings out or days off, except Sunday mornings to go to church. Adults and children worked as one, woven into a community of intense agricultural purpose. Of course, there were songs and dances and stories at night. And there was love and kinship. Everyone's survival depended upon it.

Survival also depended upon the skill of the farm's manager—the reeve—especially when times were hard. And times had never been harder, at least not in living memory, than they became in 1348 when John Ronewyk took over as the reeve of Farnham. By this time, everyone at Farnham had heard of the terrifying "Great Mortality" that was sweeping across the mainland of Europe. And although it struck first at the English coast, it eventually reached the inland farms of southeast England. The response of the English populace was varied, similar to what Boccaccio described in Italy. Some people tried to fend off death with prudence and social distancing. Others fled to more isolated areas...taking the plague with them and infecting the countryfolk.

In a majority of places—including afflicted England as well as the European mainland—there was abject chaos and a complete breakdown of social order. Riots in the cities, along with looting and brigandry on the roads and farms. Many towns were eventually abandoned, some permanently, and many estates fell to ruin. The frightened folk who had populated them either fled or died, perishing as often by violence as by the plague. Many farm workers panicked as well—abandoning their farms, slaughtering or abandoning their animals, and sometimes slaughtering each other in frenzies of scapegoating and fear.

People who worked on estates like Farnham were especially vulnerable to both disease and crime. They had no militia or other means of armed defense, and they were less defended than ever with the breakdown of social order. Worse still, these were the least educated working people in English society and so they were vulnerable to rumor, confusion, and panic. They were people of strong Catholic faith, but that faith included tales of Satan and demons as well as God and angels. And it wasn't as if they had nothing to fear. Death and disease were everywhere, as were the very real dangers of a social order crumbling in the face of the plague.

So here is where we must flesh out in what we know from Farnham's books with what we know about the nature of people, now and always...

At many farms and estates, there were outbreaks of violence, theft, chaos, and flight, along with the outbreaks of plague among the people and contagion among the animals. But at Farnham...there was peace. Yes, Farnham people did die of plague. A *lot* of Farnham people died of plague. John Ronewyk kept very careful records for the four years that he was the reeve of Farnham—specifically, from 1348 to 1352, which were the worst plague years in that region. In those four years, it is estimated from John's records that approximately 1,300 Farnham residents died of plague, representing between a third and a half of its community, depending on how many unrecorded children lived there. And these 1,300 dead people were not strangers to each other, as millions of Covid-19 victims are strangers to us. Each one of these dead people was a friend, family member, and/or co-worker to every other Farnham person. Each person who died of plague was one of the less than 3,000 people who comprised the *entire social world* for the Farnham folks. This was a collective nightmare that we can barely comprehend.

And yet, there was something about the way John managed his farm that persuaded his people to continue to work and dwell peacefully in their little community. We know that John could not have used threats or force to keep them at Farnham, because we know that those tactics didn't work at all during the Black Death. Threats and coercion are precisely what led to the Peasants' Revolt of 1381. It must have been something else John did that convinced his people to choose peace, to choose whatever life was left to be lived, to choose whatever humanity was left to them in the midst of this inhuman nightmare of contagion and death.

From the very factual records that John kept for the successful business that he managed for the landowner, we know that the folks in the Farnham village must have farmed their land, must have husbanded their animals, must have mended their buildings, must have buried their dead...and then carried on. We know that they must have cared for each other even as they buried their dead, because the emotional integrity of their community was essential for its survival. Many of them *did* die. But no one seems to have panicked. Instead, they focused on life and on each other, and in doing so, they maintained a state of relative calm and security to the end of those "years of wonder" (which is what English medievals called their years of plague). And the Farnham community was far from the only one of its kind, because life carried on in many places through the Black Death, both in England and elsewhere. But Farnham is the community for which we have a precise and reliable record, so we know for sure that the Farnham folks and John Ronewyk *did* accomplish this remarkable feat.

Procopius offers us a model of consciousness and compassion in his narrative of the Justinian plague. Similarly, the story of John Ronewyk and his Farnham folk, derived from the records that John meticulously kept through the worst of the plague in England, offers us a model of the human capacity to keep calm and carry on, with peace and purpose, even when one's world has inexplicably become a living (and dying) hell. We will never know exactly how John and his people accomplished this act of redemption for themselves, but there is an undeniable heroism in this story about steady perseverance in the face of pandemic catastrophe. And that example can be redemptive for us all.

A Story from the Post-Columbian Plural Pandemic in the Americas

This story begins long before the Black Death released its fearsome grip on humanity, and that is only a small part of its terrible truth. We have already seen that the years from 1492 to 1600 saw the introduction of over a dozen pathogens that were novel to the peoples of the New World, and the resulting tolls of disease and death were literally beyond count. To revisit the searing observation by the historian William Denevan, the plural pandemics of the post-Columbian Americas were "possibly the greatest demographic disaster in the history of the world."[85]

The effects of that pathogenic firestorm were compounded by the hideous abuse that was inflicted on the indigenous Americans by the Spanish conquistadors, added to a pervasive drought in the middle of the 16th century, and possibly a pandemic of a hemorrhagic virus the Aztecs called "cocoliztli." Cocoliztli was endemic to the New World peoples, but it was exacerbated by the unspeakable oppression and plural pandemics that were inflicted upon them by the Spanish immigrants from the Old World. As I have said before (but this is a statistic that deserves repetition), it is estimated that approximately 56 million New World people died in the hundred years after Columbus made land with his Old World cargos, and those 56 million people represented between 85% and 95% of the people who were living in the New World in 1491. In the Annals of the Cakchiquels, we are given this painful account of the New World deaths:

85. Denevan, William M. *The Native Population of the Americas in 1492.* Madison, WI: University of Wisconsin Press, 1992, 42. Project MUSE: muse.jhu.edu/book/8750

The ancients and the father died alike,
and the stench was such that men died of it alone.
Half the people threw themselves into the ravines,
And the dogs and foxes lived the bodies of the men.
The fear of death destroyed the old people,
and the oldest son of the king
died at the same time as his young brother.

Thus did we become poor, O my children,
and thus did we survive, being only little children.
And we children were all that remained![86]

It is impossible for any of us to comprehend the agony that the New World inhabitants suffered through this cataclysm, and not just in their afflicted bodies. Imagine that at least seven out of every ten people you know will perish horribly within your own life, dying with no comprehension of their misery other than some shameful misconceptions about what had caused this conflagration of suffering. Specifically, imagine that you and your people, encouraged by the new oppressors in your land, believe that you are being punished by angry gods for your bad behavior or evil character. And the details of your sins remain unnamed, but you know they must be heinous, given the extremity of your "punishments." It was not only the physical existence of the New World people that was in peril during this hideous century. It was their shining spirit as well.

It could easily have been the case that we would possess no enduring record of these accomplished, intelligent, powerful, and passionate peoples, aside from the racist accounts of their Spanish oppressors. But there was one man whose steadfast devotion and inexplicable courage defied the forces—political, pragmatic, religious, and biologic—that were arrayed against the indigenous peoples. One man who was able to compose an incredible memorial to at least one group of the New World nations...the Aztec peoples of what we now call Mexico.

His name was Bernardino de Sahagún, and he was a young Franciscan friar who came to "New Spain" in 1529 with the second group of Franciscan

86. Xajilâ, Francisco H. A. and Francisco Rojas. *The Annals of the Cakchiquels.* Translated by Daniel Brinton. Philadelphia: Gutenberg Press, 1574/1885/2005, 171. https://www.google.com/books/edition/The_Annals_of_the_Cakchiquels/HduyIgfPhyMC?hl=en&gbpv=0

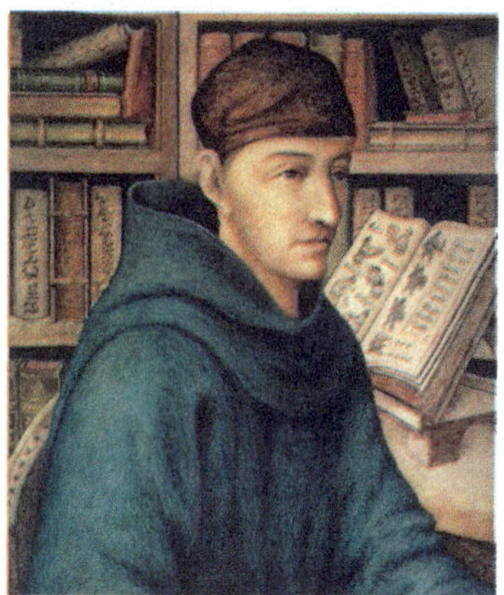

Bernardino de Sahagún, 1499-1590 (Wikimedia)

priests whose goal it was to share their Christian faith with the peoples of the New World. These Franciscan missionaries were distinctly different from most of their racist peers, and indeed, they were more enlightened than the many ethnocentric missionaries in our own era. The Franciscans of the early 16th century were convinced that the newly discovered peoples of the New World would cleanse the Old World of its spiritual corruption by incorporating their fresh faith and natural ways into the rigidified dogma and putrefied practices that the Franciscans detested in the Roman Catholic Church.

For these reasons, Bernardino was determined to learn all he could from the native peoples in this novel land so that he and his brethren could blend their own beliefs with those of the native Americans and celebrate a renewed form of Christian faith. In addition to these intercultural aspirations, Bernardino possessed a prodigious linguistic talent that greatly supported his goals, enabling him to learn at least five of the languages (or dialects) of the Aztec people.

But the most remarkable thing about Bernardino (and this quality would remain remarkable amongst *all* scholars who want to study other cultures, even to the present day) was that he wanted to see the Aztec people *through Aztec eyes*. For this reason, he interviewed Aztec people of all ages and occupations, including both men *and* women. He asked them about every aspect of their lives and specialties of work. Sometimes Bernardino let his discussants carry the conversation in whatever directions they wanted, and sometimes he guided the interview with structured questions, especially when concrete information was necessary (about the sciences, for example).

Bernardino spoke with them in their own language, and then *he wrote down* ***everything*** *they said*. He phonetically transcribed their spoken dialects of Nahuatl into Latin script, and he later translated it all into Spanish, so that other Spaniards could see the Aztec world as the Aztecs saw it. In addition, Bernardino asked the Aztec artists to create images of the things they were describing, everything from the plants and animals of their lands to the occupations they practiced and the gods they worshipped. Some images were black and white drawings, but most were illuminated with the rich colors in the native style.[87]

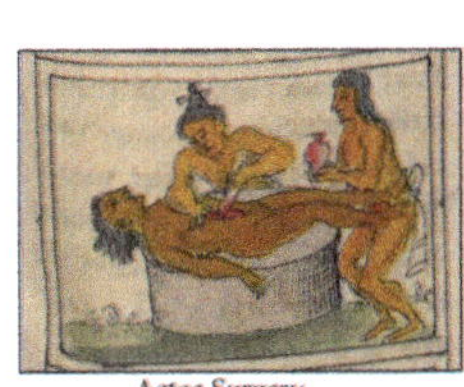
Aztec Surgery

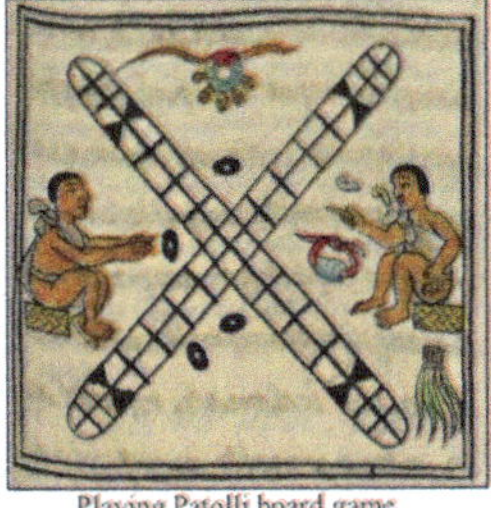
Playing Patolli board game

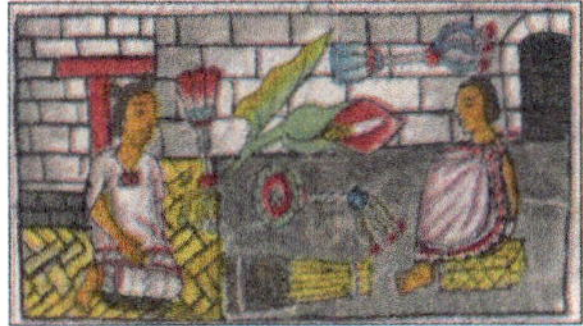
Perfume maker at work

All from *Historia General* (Wikimedia)

In the end, Bernardino and his students spent 61 years, until his death in 1590 at the age of 91, compiling all of this information into one remarkable volume. In this book, the handwritten Nahuatl and Spanish texts appear side by side (using Bernardino's rendering of Nahuatl into Latin script), and the relevant images are placed nearby. He called this enormous volume of work *Historia General De Las Cosas De La Nueva España* (*General History of the Things of New Spain*). Its final length was 2,400 pages.

It is a miracle that we know anything about this astonishing accomplishment, because by the time Bernardino completed his chronicle of the Aztec world, the Spanish Inquisition was raging—in Mexico as well as in Europe. Had the Inquisitors learned about the full scope of Bernardino's work, they would have deemed his granting of such respect to native views and practices to be an act of heresy, punishable by torture, certainly, and possibly even by death.

To avoid these punishments, Bernardino sent copies of the less inflammatory pages from his book to the Spanish court, as evidence that he was not in violation of the laws of the Church and his country. He hid from the Church his Nahuatl translations of the Psalms and a catechism, translations that would have been viewed as mortal sin. This bought a bit of time for Bernardino and the Aztecs, but the Inquisition accelerated to such a degree that, between 1570 and 1575, all religious works in Nahuatl were banned by the Church, and Bernardino was ordered to relinquish to the Inquisitors his entire volume of research. He did comply with their

87. *Florentine Codex: General History of the Things of New Spain* (Translation of and Introduction to *Historia General de Las Cosas de La Nueva España;* 12 Volumes in 13 Books). Bernardino de Sahagún, Translated by Charles E. Dibble and Arthur J. O Anderson. Salt Lake City: University of Utah Press, 1950-1982.

order...but only after he had made two more copies of the entire 2,400-page *Historia General.*

Bernardino became deeply disillusioned with the Church's mission of "spiritual conquest" in the face of the Inquisition's suppression of his work and their oppression of his beloved Aztec people. He devoted the rest of his life to an attempt to preserve the school of higher education that he had helped develop for Aztec youth in 1540—the Colegio de Santa Cruz de Tlatelolco. The school did not survive the repressive forces of the Inquisition and Spanish imperialism, but Bernardino's work of documentation *did* survive...inexplicably and, indeed, rather miraculously.

It is amazing enough that Bernardino was able to avoid prosecution by the Inquisitors. But far more astonishing is the fact that he was able, through a process that will remain forever cloaked in mystery, to convey his remaining two copies of *Historia General* into safekeeping. After Bernardino's death, those two copies of his massive book *disappeared for two centuries.* They were only discovered in 1791, when a bibliographer identified them during a random inventory of the Laurentian Library in Florence, Italy. To this day, no one knows how they got there.

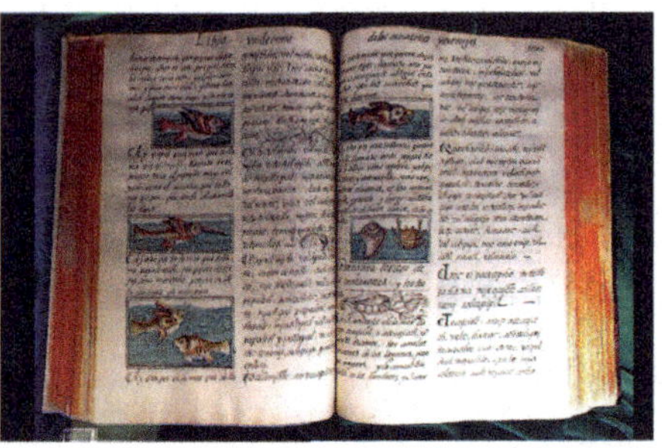

Historia General De Las Cosas De La Nueva España (The Florentine Codex) Bernardino de Sahagún, (1570). Biblioteca Medicea-Laurenziana, Florence, Italy (Wikimedia)

One hundred and fifty years after the discovery of those copies in Italy, two American scholars—Arthur J.O. Anderson and Charles Dibble—spent 30 more years translating the entire *Historia General* into English, employing the 19th century practices of Mexican scholars Francisco del Paso y Troncoso and Joaquin Garcia Icazbalceta. In 1950, Anderson and Dibble published their translation under its current title in the English-speaking world—*The Florentine Codex.*[88]

Technically, there are over thirty surviving codices that contain pictorial records from the Aztec world, but few make reference to Aztec life before

88. *Florentine Codex: General History of the Things of New Spain* (Translation of and Introduction to *Historia General de Las Cosas de La Nueva España;* 12 Volumes in 13 Books). Bernardino de Sahagún, Translated by Charles E. Dibble and Arthur J. O Anderson. Salt Lake City: University of Utah Press, 1950-1982.

the Spanish invasion.[89] In this context, Bernardino's creation of *Historia General* is an astounding accomplishment. Not only is it a comprehensive portrait of an ancient and complex culture that was entirely novel to its writer, but it was created with the intent of describing that culture from the perspective of the culture's own people. This practice, which we now call "ethnography," is still a challenging undertaking, and even its modern practitioners are not always able to achieve the degree of immersion and fidelity that Bernardino and his collaborators seemed to have attained in their massive tome.

But more than that, it is crucial to remember that Bernardino was creating the *Historia General* during the same century when it is estimated that 85 to 95% of the Aztec people (like all Native Americans) were dying from a combination of the pandemic diseases that the Europeans had brought to the Americas and the brutal treatments inflicted on them by the conquistadors. This means that the whole time Bernardino was composing the Codex, he was also watching the plural pandemics and Spanish oppression decimate the Aztec people—people whom he believed were integral to the return of Jesus Christ, people whom he had esteemed enough to interview and collaborate with for sixty years, people who had likely become his friends as well as his colleagues.

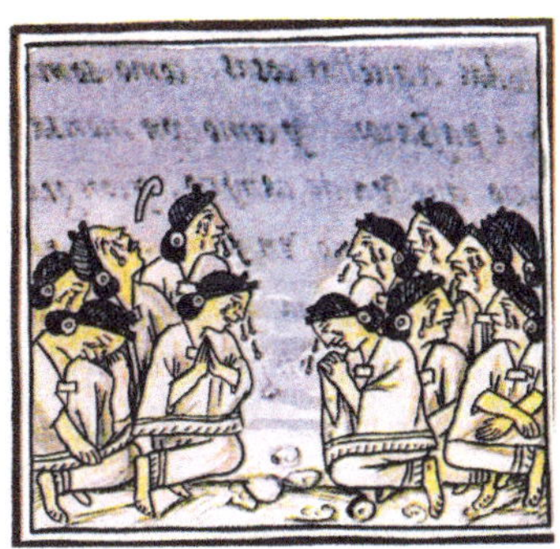

"Mourning the dead,"
The Florentine Codex (Wikimedia)

In the records left by Procopius, Boccaccio, and John Ronewyk, we have seen three narratives created by individuals who believed their worlds were literally dying, when those worlds were actually undergoing deep transformations. But in the case of the Aztecs whom Bernardino was describing, a known world and its people were dying very literally—both culturally and biologically—and they were dying while Bernardino recorded, transcribed, translated, and compiled their story. He was helpless to save the Aztecs. He could only save their memory.

There is no way to fully comprehend and honor what was lost when the Aztec peoples, like most New World peoples, succumbed to the plural pandemics and cultural genocide that transpired in the post-Columbian Americas. Nonetheless, Bernardino de Sahagún spent his life composing

89. https://en.wikipedia.org/wiki/Aztec_codices

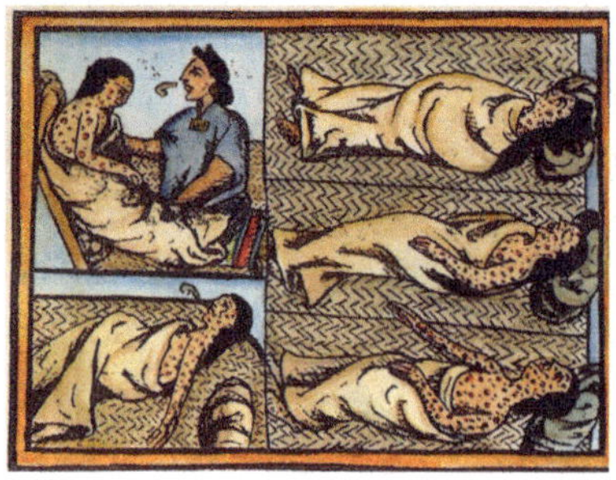

"Dying of the small pox," *The Florentine Codex* (Wikimedia)

a narrative that has miraculously survived to memorialize the Aztecs' story, including their vibrant lives, their rich culture, their unspeakable suffering, and their incomprehensible loss. If one cannot save a world, at least one can memorialize it with a narrative of devotion and respect.

A Narrative of the 1918 Flu Epidemic

Before we can say anything about the consensual narrative of the 1918 flu epidemic, we must first revisit its facts, as best they have been estimated by reputable historians and demographers. In 1918, the world's methods of recording illness and death were nearly prehistoric by comparison to ours, but we can say with some confidence that approximately one half of the world's population—which totaled 1.8 billion in 1918—contracted *influenza H1N1.* And of the approximately 900 million people who contracted the flu, at least 50 million people died of either the flu or its secondary infections such as pneumonia. (No antibiotics, remember?) And most of this disease and death happened within the space of eighteen months.

In other words, the influenza epidemic of 1918-19 killed more people, and faster, than any other event in human history. That is noteworthy in itself. But the truly astonishing fact is that this viral firestorm left nearly no trace on our collective memory. No consensual narrative. Barely any narrative at all, really. The story was to arrive later—*much* later—than its facts. So our first task, before we can select a narrative for the 1918 flu epidemic, is to consider the possible reasons for this bewildering blind spot in our collective consciousness.

Whatever one can say about the three pandemics we have already visited in this chapter, what we can*not* say is that they went unnoticed by those who suffered and died in them, nor were they lightly dismissed by those who were fortunate enough to survive and reflect upon them. We don't have a lot of documentation that survives from the 6th, 14th, and 16th centuries, but what documentation we *do* have makes it quite clear that the contemporary people in these pandemics were horrifically aware of the pestilential conflagrations that were burning down their worlds.

By stark contrast, the 1918 flu was virtually ignored for decades by nearly all historical accounts, except for a few medical historians. And those medical historians only mentioned the flu pandemic because they felt it was important to learn more about its deadly protagonist. Their task wasn't easy, because viruses were undetectable, and therefore undiscussable, until Richard Shope isolated the swine flu virus in 1931, and later found that antibodies to the swine flu were present in humans who had contracted the 1918 flu. So to some degree, the lack of scientific discussion about the 1918 flu was the result of its virus's literal invisibility until 1933.

But that doesn't explain the absence of discussion about the *consequences* of H1N1's deadly rampage around the world. There were, after all, at least 50 million dead people to bury or burn—people who had surely meant *something* to the people they left behind. And those who survived the flu often had long-lasting disabilities from its ravages, not to mention the posttraumatic psychological effects of living through the pandemic. However, even after Shope's crucial identification of the *influenza A* virus in the mid-1930s, the printing presses remained oddly silent on the subject of the 1918 pandemic. And not just silent for a year or two, while people recovered from the trauma of a global war. They were *silent for 50 years after the end of the pandemic.* The medical historian Howard Phillips had this to say in 2004 about those strangely silent fifty years—half a century that was virtually devoid of publication about the 1918 flu pandemic:

> "What is [most] remarkable...is the almost complete silence of professional historians of the day about the pandemic, in striking contrast to their readiness to tackle as a historical topic its contemporary, World War I. Although they had lived through both, it was almost as if they deemed a world war to be suitable as a subject for historians but not a world pandemic."[90]

With few exceptions, this is how things remained in both the professional and public presses—silence on the subject of the worst pandemic die-off in human history. It was an inexplicable silence that began to be broken, very quietly, one day in 1968. This was the day I've already alluded to—the day when the young history professor Alfred Crosby was in the library of Washington State University, digging through materials from 1918 in his study of the losses suffered as a result of the soldiers killed in World War I. The more deeply Professor Crosby dug, the more it became clear that the

90. Phillips, Howard. "The Re-appearing Shadow of 1918: Trends in the Historiography of the 1918-19 Influenza Pandemic." *Canadian Bulletin of Medical History*, Volume 21:1 (2004), p. 121-134

losses suffered as a result of the war were overwhelmingly eclipsed by the losses suffered as a result of the influenza epidemic...an epidemic that Crosby had always seen relegated to footnotes and sidebars about that period.

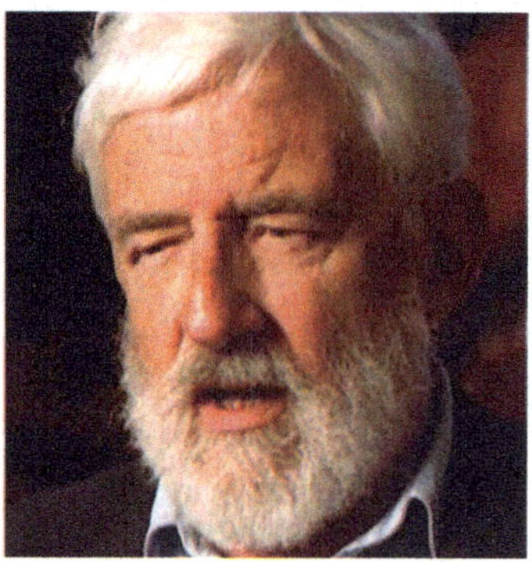

Professor Alfred W. Crosby (Still photo from 1997 video aired in 2009 on PBS/ WGBH)

We are fortunate that Professor Crosby was not only brilliant and disciplined, but he also possessed a far-reaching knowledge base and a mind attuned to insight and explanation, particularly on the effect of biological forces in historic events. Crosby had already published a book on what he called "the Columbian exchange"—a landmark concept in which he had identified the biological factors of historic human contacts (including contagious diseases) that previous scholars had ignored, despite the fact that those factors had profoundly influenced key interactions among various peoples throughout world history.[91]

Therefore, when Crosby stumbled upon the blazing statistics of morbidity and mortality from the 1918 flu, he immediately recognized that the forces of biological imperative had trounced the forces of human aggression. (Yes, human aggression was far more feared in 1918, as it is today, even though it turned out to be far less deadly than the flu.) In 1976, Crosby returned to the publishing house that had bravely put forth his book on "the Columbian exchange," and he persuaded them to publish his book on the even more obscure topic of the 1918 flu pandemic. He entitled this second book *Epidemic and Peace, 1918.*[92]

Over the next few years, Crosby's work evolved and expanded in the direction of his first book, which led to the publication of a third book, again on the subject of "the Columbian exchange," a subject for which he was to acquire renown among historians.[93] But during the 1980s, while Professor Crosby was deepening his work on the role of biology in cultural domination, a different kind of biological domination was occurring around the globe in the realm of the human immune system. A new pandemic

91. Crosby, Alfred W. *The Columbian Exchange: Biological and Cultural Consequences of 1492.* Westport, CN: Greenwood Press, 1972.

92. Crosby, Alfred W. *Epidemic and Peace, 1918.* Westport, CN: Greenwood Press, 1976.

93. Crosby, Alfred W. *Ecological Imperialism: The biological Expansion of Europe, 900-1900.* Cambridge, MA: Cambridge University Press, 1986, 1993, 2004.

invader was waging a campaign of world conquest, and it was racking up a frightening number of victims. The name of the new micro-invader was Human Immunodeficiency Virus, traveling under the nickname HIV, and it was accompanied by its morbid offspring, Acquired Immune Deficiency Syndrome, whose street tag was the dread diagnosis AIDS.[94]

Humankind had wrestled with various disease outbreaks since 1918, including several bouts with the descendants of *influenza H1N1* (although we didn't know they were its descendants at the time). But most Americans were far more attentive to the medical victories of the mid-20th century, partly as a result of advances in medical treatments (yes, including antibiotics), and partly as a result of the myriad advances in the field of vaccination. Take a look at this list of release dates for vaccines that we now consider to be essential preparations for a healthy life:

Yellow fever	1938
Influenza	1945
Diphtheria	1948
Tetanus	1948
Pertussis	1948
Polio	1955
Measles	1963
Mumps	1967
Rubella	1969
Chickenpox	1988

And then came HIV/AIDS. Suddenly, we were faced with a deadly pandemic disease that had no known means of prevention or cure. We hadn't been confronted with such a lethal monster since...well...1918. Although some (perhaps many) of us retreated into regrettable postures of denial, projection, and magical thinking in response to HIV/AIDS, others of us thought it might be a good idea to follow George Santayana's advice and learn from the past so that we would not be condemned to repeat it. We looked back at other deadly pandemics, particularly those that involved incurable and deadly viruses, and particularly pandemics of relatively recent memory. And there we rediscovered Alfred Crosby's book about the 1918 flu pandemic. In 1989, when the

94. Although I have not included the AIDS pandemic in this book, I would like to cite as a worthy consensual narrative of the AIDS epidemic Larry Kramer's play *The Normal Heart* (1985, New York, NY: Samuel French, Inc. and the related 2014 HBO film). Equal endorsement goes to Randy Shilts' *And the Band Played On* (1993, HBO).

AIDS epidemic was really beginning to terrify Americans, the esteemed Cambridge University Press republished Crosby's *Epidemic and Peace, 1918* under a snazzy new title: *America's Forgotten Pandemic: The Influenza of 1918*. Suddenly, what had been long forgotten was newly remembered.[95]

And so it was that Americans were awakened, with much amazement, to the power of microscopic natural forces in the determination of human events. Certainly, we had already come to suspect that small actions with environmental consequences could have large implications for future generations. But too many decades had passed since our last encounter with the world-changing power of pandemic disease, and we had forgotten whatever lessons we might have learned...if we had ever learned them in the first place. HIV/AIDS sent us running back to the old 1918 flu (much as the novel coronavirus has recently done), where we hoped to find some insight into this infinitesimal new enemy that was mowing us down with such audacity.

The answers that Alfred Crosby offered us about that previous infinitesimal enemy—an invader that had mowed us down more than 80 years before, in even greater numbers, and with even greater speed—were as sobering as they were complex. There was a wealth of knowledge and insight to be gained from Crosby's book, but little of it was comforting. For one thing, Crosby observed that the 1989 public's confidence in science was now in crisis:

> Scientists know amazingly more about molecular biology, pathogens, and immunology than they did fifteen or twenty years ago, but the bad guys, the pathogens, particularly the newly recognized ones, seem to the general public to have become nastier, faster than the scientists have become smarter.[96]

But more than that, there was the larger phenomenon of the invisibility of the 1918 pandemic to our collective eyes, both during the period it had occurred and during the decades since it had mysteriously subsided:

> [The 1918 influenza] inspires anxiety and confusion in us—anxiety because it was so awful and we do not know why, and confusion because we cannot understand how we could have so nearly forgotten it.[97]

95. Crosby, Alfred W. *America's Forgotten Pandemic: The Influenza of 1918*. New York: Cambridge University Press, 1989, 2003.

96. Ibid. page xi.

97. Ibid. page xiv.

Some of the flu's invisibility in our memory may have been a result of the sampling bias (remember that?) that humanity is always inclined to display when it comes to pandemic disease. Crosby described it this way, and much more poetically than the social psychologists:

> [God], jaded with omnipotence, seems to have posed Himself a paradoxical problem; just how deadly a disease can I create that humans will barely notice? The answer to His challenge was influenza... On the whole, we humans are more frightened of diseases with high mortality rates which we are *not* apt to get, than of diseases with low but quite real mortality rates which we are almost certain to get eventually.[98]

So a crucial part of the 1918 flu narrative must include the facts that 1) we had never understood its lethality to begin with, 2) we continued to underestimate its power even after it had killed us by the millions, and most incomprehensibly of all, 3) we seemed to have forgotten about it entirely once it departed. Not that we forgot about the flu in a *personal* sense, because we know that *individual* people didn't forget about the flu and its deadly consequences. But American *society* forgot, or else ignored, the cataclysm of contagion and death that H1N1 brought down upon us. And so did the rest of the world, by the way.

Well, putting aside for a moment the consensual narrative of H1N1, let's start with the facts—the skeleton inside this beast of a story—the facts that we have briefly visited in this book:

Our protagonist in the 1918 drama originated inside a Kansas chicken (well, probably a bunch of Kansas chickens), and then it jumped the species fence to a Kansas pig, where it acquired the pathogenic clout that made it such a pandemic superstar. Then it seems to have jumped the species fence again, in March 1918, to an army cook in Fort Funston, Kansas. After that, it quickly hitched a ride with the war troops to Europe, and soon after, it made a barn-burning world tour, beginning with Africa and South America, and eventually traveling to Asia and every corner of the globe.

The pandemic transpired in four waves. The first lasted through the spring and early summer of 1918, and that wave was the least deadly of the three. Then, beginning in August 1918, the second wave of influenza began and it incinerated every population it touched. For example, in just the *last*

98. Ibid. page xiv.

three months of 1918, the flu killed 300,000 Americans (which would be the equivalent of about 1.2 million Americans in today's population). It was even deadlier in India, exploding India's death toll to somewhere between *12 and 20 million deaths during those same three months*. The third wave of the pandemic occurred in the first six months of 1919, and although the numbers of sick and dead were still staggering, they were less than in the second wave, possibly because more people had acquired immunity from having been sick. The fourth wave of flu occurred in the spring of 1920, and although some areas were missed altogether, the areas that had been lightly touched in previous waves suffered terribly during this final surge.

There is still controversy about how many people were infected and/or killed by *influenza H1N1*, because it is impossible to extract precise numbers from locations that are so distant from us in culture and time. But once again, averaging across the historians' arguments, the conservative estimate remains at 900 million people infected and 50 million killed. This means that approximately 50% of the world's population became sick with this flu, and it killed approximately 5% of the people in the world. This may not seem like such a catastrophe when compared to the kill rate of the plural pandemic in the post-Columbian age, but remember that most of these 50 million people *died within 18 months*, as compared to 100 years. Corpses were piled in the streets of Philadelphia and other major cities. Health systems were overwhelmed and local governments were in chaos when faced with the challenges of managing the contagion and its consequences.

Clearly, it wasn't as if no one knew that the pandemic was happening during the time it was infecting and killing people. It was just happening too fast and too confoundingly for anyone to do much that was effective, or even clarifying. And then this killer version of the flu vanished, almost as suddenly as it had arrived. The disaster was simply too mind-boggling for anyone to really comprehend it...and therefore, too confounding for anyone to really memorialize it.

In addition, it should be noted that there were a variety of large coincidences which both amplified and obscured the power of this pandemic protagonist. There was a major climate anomaly in Europe that produced cold, wet weather beyond all norms.[99] This meant that the environmental conditions for the troops and civilians in World War I were a perfect soup

99. More, Alexander F., Christopher P. Loveluck, Heather Clifford, Michael J. Handley, Elena V. Korotkikh, Andrei V. Kurbatov, et al. "The impact of a six-year climate anomaly on the "Spanish flu" pandemic and WWI" *GeoHealth*. 4 (9) (September 2020) https://doi.org/10.1029/2020GH000277

of opportunity for any pathogen—crowded, filthy, damp, exhausting, constantly migrating, and extremely stressful.

But perhaps most helpful of all to *influenza H1N1* was the incessant, insidious, and ruthless drama of World War I itself. All war is filthy and despicable, but WWI was by all accounts extreme in both those elements. Conducted in a swamp of mud by soldiers who were ill-equipped and unprotected, little more than grist for the relentless mill of chaotic combat, WWI was the ideal petri dish for breeding a pandemic superweapon—a pathogen with unprecedented contagion and lethality. People at war and at home were infected and dying so fast that it was impossible to track them all, and the demands of the war kept those infected people on the move within their regions and around the world. It was a viral firestorm unlike any that humankind had ever seen.

When we humans see something that we have never seen before, and especially when we see it while something noisier and more familiar (like a war) is occurring simultaneously, it is both tempting and convenient to devote our entire attention, and our enduring memory, to the larger and noisier object. And this, it appears, is what we did—we Americans and, more generally, we humans. The story of the 1918 flu pandemic was devoured and absorbed by our consensual narrative for World War I. It became a sad little subplot to the gargantuan saga of what we were proudly calling "the war to end all wars." This epithet seems tragically deluded now, but it probably boosted the morale of those who spoke it during the war, and it certainly depicts the awe with which the American public regarded its first-ever *world* war. How globally important we Americans must have felt!

> Over there, over there,
> Send the word, send the word over there
> That the Yanks are coming, the Yanks are coming
> The drums rum-tumming everywhere.
> So prepare, say a prayer,
> Send the word, send the word to beware –
> We'll be over, we're coming over,
> And we won't come back till it's over, over there.[100]

100. Cohan, George M. "Over There!" New York: Leo Feist, Inc., 1917.

With all of this war-time glory (and that sense of glory applied to the European allies and the Germans as well as the "Yanks"), how could we give much credence to a "little bird whose name was Enza," a "bad cold" that many people referred to casually as "the Spanish lady"? This was no time to lay in bed and let the "Huns" win the war! This was the time to be tough, to keep our chins up and our eyes fixed on a triumphant horizon. So we marched forth...into the stuffy barracks, into the seething troop ships, into the poorly ventilated war factories, into the stinking trenches. And we got sick. And lot of us died. Or else we passed the virus along to many others, with an estimated R (contagion) factor that was possibly double or triple what the coronavirus entails.

The *real* winner of World War I was *influenza H1N1.* All the deluded notions that obscure that fact might explain our lack of a consensual narrative about the 1918 flu pandemic. Specifically, as long as we turned our backs on the overwhelming lethality of the flu, we could continue to claim and believe that *we* had won that awful war! To preserve our glorious narrative of World War I, we erased all narratives of the flu. Or at least, we erased all *consensual* narratives.

At the end of his remarkable book, Alfred Crosby has this to say, and it is a sentiment that has since been echoed by other writers: [101]

> As one searches for explanations for the odd fact that Americans took little notice of the pandemic, and then quickly forgot whatever they did notice, one comes upon a mystery and a paradox. Americans [in general] barely noticed and didn't recall... But if one turns to intimate accounts...if one asks those who lived through the pandemic for their reminiscences, then it becomes apparent that Americans *did* notice, Americans were frightened, the courses of their lives were deflected into new channels...they remember the pandemic quite clearly and often acknowledge it as one of the most influential experiences of their lives... [The flu] had a permanent influence not on the collectivities but on the *atoms* of human society—individuals.[102]

101. Outka, Elizabeth *Viral Modernism: The Influenza Pandemic and Interwar Literature .New York:* Columbia University Press, 2019.

102. Crosby, Alfred W. *America's Forgotten Pandemic: The Influenza of 1918.* New York: Cambridge University Press, 1989, 2003, pp 322-323.

That "atomized" effect of the 1918 flu was not only evident in America, and it was perhaps most clearly evident in the post-war work of many creative writers. The Irish poet William Butler Yeats was profoundly affected by the flu, especially after his wife George contracted the virus during her pregnancy and nearly died along with their unborn child. Through her convalescence, Yeats wrote these words to commemorate the threatened disintegration of their known world, both socially and biologically:

> Turning and turning in the widening gyre
> The falcon cannot hear the falconer;
> Things fall apart; the centre cannot hold;
> Mere anarchy is loosed upon the world,
> The blood-dimmed tide is loosed, and everywhere
> The ceremony of innocence is drowned;
> The best lack all conviction, while the worst
> Are full of passionate intensity.
>
> Surely some revelation is at hand;
> Surely the Second Coming is at hand.
> The Second Coming! Hardly are those words out
> When a vast image out of *Spiritus Mundi*
> Troubles my sight: somewhere in sands of the desert
> A shape with lion body and the head of a man,
> A gaze blank and pitiless as the sun,
> Is moving its slow thighs, while all about it
> Reel shadows of the indignant desert birds.
> The darkness drops again; but now I know
> That twenty centuries of stony sleep
> Were vexed to nightmare by a rocking cradle,
> And what rough beast, its hour come round at last,
> Slouches towards Bethlehem to be born?[103]

In a similar vein, we find what is possibly the best novel describing the flu pandemic, a novel written by an author of that post-WWI period. The novel is *Pale Horse Pale Rider*, written by Katherine Anne Porter, who suffered both from the flu herself and from the tragic loss of a loved one who died

103. Yeats, William Butler. "The Second Coming" in *The Norton Anthology of Modern and Contemporary Poetry.* New York: W.W. Norton, 1919/2003.

of the flu. Based closely upon her own experience, Porter's story recounts the anguish of Miranda, a newspaper reporter who is stricken by influenza at the same time as her beloved Adam, a soldier in the war. Miranda nearly dies of the flu, temporarily losing her hair and the use of her leg. Eventually, she does recover...only to learn that Adam has died of the disease. Porter's descriptions of the era are precise and piercing. But it is the ending of her story that conveys the legacy of *influenza H1N1* in the bodies and hearts of those who survived its scourge:

> No more war, no more plague, only the dazed silence that follows the ceasing of heavy guns; noiseless houses with the shades drawn, empty streets, the dead cold light of tomorrow. Now there would be time for everything.[104]

In the end, it seems that when we seek a consensual narrative for the 1918 flu pandemic, we must rely upon artists to convey the essence of a story that most human minds could not comprehend or contain. The flu struck too fast, too lethally, and too mysteriously, and it departed too suddenly for anyone to metabolize the global terror and grief it left behind.

The influenza pandemic burned through the world when Albert Camus was only six years old, but it obviously left a searing impression on his psyche. When Camus was criticized for his choice to write a novel about a subject as morbid as the plague, Camus responded that it seemed "entirely natural" to him. And at the same time, we know that Camus also felt that "a pestilence is not a thing made to man's measure." In *The Plague,* Camus expresses the belief that humanity, when faced with forces enormously larger than itself, cannot take responsibility for the superhuman situation, but we can (and should) take responsibility for how we respond to it.[105]

The artistic remnants from the flu pandemic convey the "atomic" essence of the consensual narrative that Alfred Crosby began to assemble for us in 1968, when he himself awakened to the collective magnitude of the 1918 pandemic. To quote Crosby once again:

> Nothing else—no infection, no war, no famine—has ever killed so many in as short a period. And yet it has never inspired

104. Porter, Katherine Anne. "Pale Horse Pale Rider" in *The Collected Stories of Katherine Anne Porter.* New York: Harcourt Brace, 1965, pp 269-317.

105. Camus, Albert. *The Plague (La Peste).* New York: Vintage, 1939/1965.

> awe, not in 1918 and not since, not among the citizens of any particular land, and certainly not among the citizens of the United States.[106]

Even from the perspective of this astute historian, the narrative of the 1918 flu pandemic may forever reside, as it always has, in myriad traces of individual suffering, courage, despair, and reminiscence. Grief of this magnitude may, in fact, be collectively unspeakable, leaving us to scour among these deathless mementoes—memorial embers that linger for us to rediscover, reignite, and revere.

A Narrative of the Novel Coronavirus Pandemic

If there is anything more difficult than telling a story that has been ignored and forgotten, it is to tell a story that has not yet revealed its ending—a story that has not yet even revealed its essential form.

All we have in the way of a narrative for the coronavirus pandemic is a collage of events from the short time since the pandemic formally slapped our collective consciousness in the face. Nowhere has this collage of events appeared as a consensual narrative, but it has appeared as a collage of words, spare but elegant, composed by Anthony Faiola of *The Washington Post*.[107] Let's contemplate that collage and embellish it with what we have learned thus far about humanity's global pandemics.

We have seen from the four preceding narratives that every pandemic evokes a host of competing contrasts. Courage competes with terror. Compassion competes with self-absorption. Community competes with isolation. Survival competes with sacrifice. Truth competes with falsehood. Sometimes these contrasts erupt in violent opposition, and sometimes they simmer in quiet paradox. Life is replete with such contrasts, but never more than during a pandemic, when a microbial firebug ignites a conflagration of misery beyond all human measure. Pestilence is the first of the apocalyptic Horsemen because we fear Him the most. As well we should.

106. Crosby, Alfred W. *America's Forgotten Pandemic: The Influenza of 1918*. Cambridge, MA.: Cambridge University Press, 1989, 2003, pp 311.

107. Much of the inspiration and some of the substance for this section are gifts from the summary article by Anthony Faiola of *The Washington Post*, which he entitled "How future generations will judge humanity's performance against the coronavirus." (March 4, 2021) I offer my profound gratitude to Mr. Faiola for his breadth of vision and lovely prose, and I hope that the use I make of his creation will do credit to his work. https://www.washingtonpost.com/world/2021/03/04/global-pandemic-coronavirus-response/

Pestilence is especially terrifying to people like us—people who have had the good fortune to be protected from most epidemic disease for the whole of our lives. Decades of immunization and antiseptic procedure (thank you, Drs. Jenner and Semmelweis) have made most people in our generation, especially most American people, casually dismissive when it comes to the lethal power of the microscopic adventurers who seek new lands to conquer within our bodies.

Some of us have remained ignorant, by choice or by default, regarding the threat that those diseases pose to our vulnerable flesh. Others of us have decided that we are more powerful than those infinitesimal invaders, assuming a position of arrogance (or more charitably, overconfidence) with regard to the danger posed by pandemic disease. Ignorance and arrogance are a perilous combination under any circumstance, but especially when they co-occur in the face of a deadly threat. The pairing of ignorance and arrogance are most dangerous when they prevail in privileged First World communities, which includes most American communities, because we have the capacity to spread our potent influence throughout the world—for its redemption or ruin.

And so it was, in December 2019, that apocalyptic Pestilence galloped straight through our flimsy delusion of biological invulnerability, mounted on His white charger of viral contagion and death. He quickly began to mow us down with a blazing scythe that was, to us, both confounding and calamitous. And in doing so, Pestilence activated a host of oppositional contrasts that have become as white-hot as His horse.

For example, you have learned in this book that our immune systems have super-heated into deadly contrasts when they do battle with this truly *novel* coronavirus. Remember that disquieting term "thrombo-hemorrhagic *derangement*"? Covid-19 has thrown the human immune system into a spasm of oppositional madness that may be unprecedented in pandemic history, and the consequences are evident in the chaos of our Covid-induced symptom sets. The damages done by this novel protagonist have been more diverse than those of any other pandemic disease, but all Covid victims have one thing in common. The coronavirus chimera has seared its brand into every person it has attacked, as a consequence of the heated civil wars it has ignited in our immune systems—the bewildered micro-defenders of our tale.

The most visible contrasts, however, have appeared among the macro-defenders of this story—our human behaviors. And the contrasts in our human behaviors have also erupted into adversarial infernos. Of course, every pandemic drama of history has revealed in its human players the stress responses I described in the last chapter. But the coronavirus pandemic has made those responses, and their contrasts, starkly evident. As we attempt to compose a narrative for this pandemic, as we consider the conduct of human groups in a world infested with coronavirus, the contrasts in our response patterns must play a large role in the story. Here is where Mr. Faiola's summary of humanity's pandemic response is most applicable, so I will weave my observations into his.

China initially retreated into *denial*, minimizing to the world (and possibly to itself) the danger and degree of the contagion. Soon after, the leaders and followers in several prominent countries, including the United States, Brazil, and Russia, pursued the *regressed* notion that coronavirus was "just a flu" that would succumb to their superior defenses. They promoted the *magical thinking* that it would "go away soon" if it wasn't exaggerated by their "cowardly" opponents. Still other countries (like the U.K.) adopted a position of *repression* (and perhaps *reaction formation*), maintaining a stiff upper lip as they "sleepwalked into disaster" (to quote the English *Sunday Times*). In still other countries, there was a mix of responses. Germany initially adopted severe measures of *anticipation and preparation* and managed to "flatten the curve" of infection, only to lose that advantage when a large subset of right-wing Germans accused the moderate German leaders of weakness. Acting on a panoply of stress responses (*repression, projection,* and *displacement* among them), the German objecters held vast mask-less demonstrations against the "Corona False Alarm." And then Germany's Covid statistics exploded.

There has been no perfect recipe for minimizing the pandemic's damage. Australia and New Zealand achieved admirably low Covid numbers, accomplished in part with their rapid employment of *rational analysis* and *anticipation/preparation*, but also aided by their status as island nations. Other countries, like South Korea and Japan, invoked their long traditions of social compliance in order to achieve similar success initially, but have struggled with subsequent surges. The nations of Africa deployed their hard-won experience with lethal pandemics, combined with *anticipation/preparation* and *rational analysis*, to reach some of the lowest Covid numbers in the world. All of these success stories entailed a combination of *rational analysis, anticipation/preparation,* and creative *sublimation* in their responses.

And of course, there have also been astounding successes that were due to countless acts of individual heroism in every country. I refer here to the health care professionals and first responders who deployed immense amounts of *repression*, *reaction formation*, ironclad *humor*, and raw courage to contain the amounts of infection and death. Additionally, there are the "Usain Bolts of vaccine science"[108] whose *rational analysis* and *creative sublimation* combined to produce the vaccines we needed to train our B and T cell assassins, the best of our micro-defenders against the micro-invader. In the more personal realm of individual courage and sacrifice, there are the millions of people who stayed inside, wore masks, kept their distance, and worked and schooled from home...or else took every precaution to minimize contagion to their fellow humans when they ventured into public.

Conversely, on the other end of this global contrast, there have been many people who have rejected, demeaned, prohibited and/or violently overthrown these preventative measures, embracing instead the stress responses of *denial*, *regression*, *displacement*, *magical thinking*, and *projection*. These are the same people who are rejecting, in principle and in action, the vaccines that are humanity's only hope of regaining the discretionary lives that many of us previously enjoyed, often took for granted, and then abruptly sacrificed to save the lives of ourselves and others. It's hard to imagine a more blatant contrast than that.

In the end, according to Ashish Jha, dean of Brown University's School of Public Health (as quoted by Mr. Faiola), "There wasn't a single path out of this pandemic...it took being proactive and aggressive and—most of all—taking the virus seriously. A bunch of countries did it, and a bunch of countries just didn't."[109]

On the stage of American response, we see the drama of oppositional contrast played out in scenes that are poignantly tragic. And we are likely to perceive those tragedies more deeply as the acuity of hindsight sharpens our focus. Or possibly not. We humans like to avoid "cognitive dissonance," as I mentioned earlier, and that means that whatever bad outcomes result from our regrettable choices will not change the minds of those of us whose choices are leading to those bad outcomes. For example, at the Conservative Political Action Conference of 2021, South Dakota Governor Kristi Noem defended her refusal to enact anti-Covid protections in her state, claiming that her protocols were "among the most successful"...*even though South Dakota, at that very moment, had America's second highest per capita Covid*

108. Ibid. p 3..
109. Ibid. p 13

case rate, and its *eighth highest per capita Covid death rate.*[110] Similarly, Texas Governor Greg Abbott announced the removal of all anti-Covid measures in his state *on the same day that his state's Covid case increase was the highest in America.*[111]

And returning to the subject of those amazing vaccines...

Although the novel coronavirus has been seeded throughout the world by its most privileged human inhabitants—people with the ability to hop continents like some people might hop buses—Covid-19 has followed in the footsteps of its pandemic predecessors by treating most harshly the people who can least afford or withstand its assault...the disadvantaged and underprivileged. The people whom we call BIPOC in America—Black, Indigenous, People of Color—have been afflicted and struck down in devastating numbers, as contrasted with those who enjoy the privileges that are too often associated with lighter skin, European heritage, and multi-generational citizenship.

Similarly, the contrasts in access to medical care, public health education, and historic trust in the health care system may lead to a situation in which vaccination will become another advantage of multi-generational privilege in America (and elsewhere). And to the surprise of presumably no one, the rich have become richer and the poor have become poorer in the clutches of the novel coronavirus, deepening a contrast that was already fracturing social structures in America and elsewhere in the world. The sum of these oppositional tensions is articulated succinctly, even poetically, by Mr. Faiola:

> Despite decades of planning, cutting-edge centers for disease control, and years of experience battling smaller outbreaks in "poorer" countries, the world's wealthiest peoples...were unable or unwilling to halt what might mostly be remembered as a rich nation's virus without suffering massive casualties. In piercing prose, [we see] the lack of leadership. The failure to coordinate. The on-again, off-again lockdowns. The no lockdowns at all. The misinformation and politicization of a health crisis. The

110. Kelley, Alexandra. "Fauci vs. SD Gov. Kristi Noem: 'The Numbers Don't Lie'" *The Hill*, March 1, 2021 https://thehill.com/changing-america/well-being/prevention-cures/540985-fauci-vs-sd-gov-kristi-noem-the-numbers-dont-lie/

111. The Editorial Board of *The Washington Post.* "Greg Abbott is endangering the health of Texas and beyond." *The Washington Post*, March 2, 2021. https://www.washingtonpost.com/opinions/greg-abbott-is-endangering-the-health-of-texas-and-beyond/2021/03/02/55105860-7ba6-11eb-a976-c028a4215c78_story.html

> virus deniers and never-maskers from Missouri to Medellín who confused personal freedom with a criminal disregard for everyone else... [And] no single country, epidemiologists and health experts say, has suffered as great a failure as the United States. [112]

The contrast that lies at the root of nearly all the rest is the one that seems the least accessible to influence or reconciliation. It is a contrast of values, visions, and world views. It is a contrast that has riven American society for many years, but perhaps no more dramatically than in the last decade. The violent insurrection at the American Capitol building on January 6, 2021 is only the largest and most recent, but certainly not the deepest, example of the extent to which this contrast has polarized our culture.

The poet William Blake referred to a contrast like this as a "contrary," turning the adjective into a noun so that he could describe a contrast so fundamental and extremely polarized that it cuts to the core of human existence. A global massacre of the sort that only Pestilence can inflict is the kind of thing that brings into our personal experience, and sometimes our cultural consciousness, the "contraries" that can pull a society in opposing directions...and even pull it apart. This is when we strongly suspect that we have come to a time when, to revisit Yeats, "Things fall apart, the centre cannot hold, and mere anarchy is loosed upon the world."

This novel coronavirus pandemic has a narrative whose essence requires more time to reveal itself in order to be recounted. However, judging by the deeply disturbing oppositions we have witnessed in the pandemic's first years, it seems probable that the narrative of the coronavirus pandemic in America (and perhaps throughout the world) must include one or more of Blake's "contraries." If Blake was right about the nature of "contraries," our goal must be to find a broader view, a deeper vision, and a more expansive set of values that can span the two poles of contrast that define every "contrary." And then we must reconcile them into a larger whole.

Our best choice might be to cradle this unfinished narrative of the coronavirus pandemic in a combination of Blake's vision of the "contrary" and these words from the German poet Rainier Maria Rilke, published in the wake of the 1918 flu pandemic:

112. Ibid. p 3, 6.

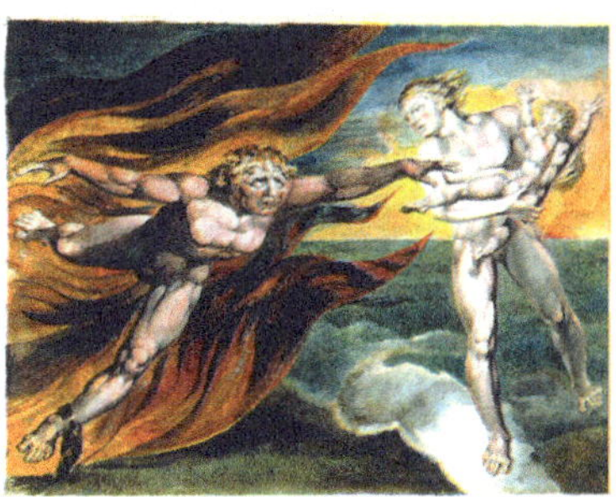

William Blake, *The Good and Evil Angels* (1795) (Wikimedia)

Take your practiced powers
and stretch them out
until they span the chasm
between two contradictions...

For the Divine wants
to know itself in you. [113]

♦ ♦ ♦

Five global pandemics, offering four consensual narratives and one suggestive collage. Upon reflection, it seems that even the best pandemic narratives can only *suggest* an essence of "tiger" from the rapacious events they describe. But if we root these narratives in their historical antecedents, and if we populate them with their key players—invaders and defenders—we obtain a felt sense of the dramas entailed in each pandemic, and in our global pandemics as a whole. Witnessing, recording, carrying on, memorializing the losses of a whole culture or a single person, torn by our "contraries" and grasping at some form of healing for soul as well as body—these are the stories of humankind in the grip of pandemic disease.

Now let us see what crude ore of meaning we can mine from such deep and dangerous journeys, and following that, what golden perspective we might refine from the raw matter of humanity's suffering. Into the fire once more...

113. Rilke, Rainer Maria. "As once the wingéd energy of delight" in *The Selected Poetry of Rainer Maria Rilke*. New York: Vintage, 1922/1948/1989.

CHAPTER 6

Some Meaningful Consequences from the Pandemics of History

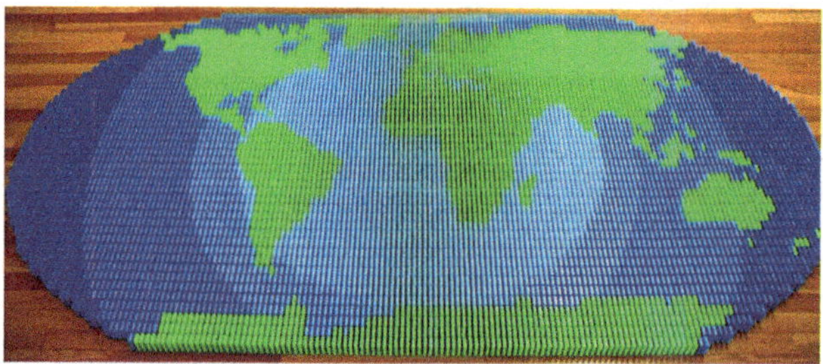

Lily Topples the World[114]

No incident, however seemingly trivial, is unimportant in the scheme of things. One event leads to another, which triggers something else and before you know where you are, the ramifications spread far and wide throughout history. Echoing down the ages. Getting fainter and fainter, but never completely dying away. They talk of The Harmony of the Spheres, but history is A Symphony of Echoes. Every little action has huge consequences... It makes your head ache.

– **Jodi Taylor,** *A Symphony of Echoes*[115]

The complexities of cause and effect defy analysis.

– **Douglas Adams,** *Dirk Gently's Holistic Detective Agency*[116]

We can't help it. No matter how colossal a story may be, we want to know what it *means.* After all is said and done, what difference has it made that this story has transpired? Every storyteller will confirm that it's a lot easier to *tell* a story—factual or fictional—than it is to name the effects that the

114. Domino art by Lily Hevesh (https://youtu.be/FWgH0hXZKrE and https://lilytopplestheworld.com/)

115. Taylor, Jodi. *A Symphony of Echoes.* New York: Night Shade Books, 2015.

116. Adams, Douglas. *Dirk Gently's Holistic Detective Agency.* New York: Pocket Books, 1987.

story has had on the things that follow. Now, it is true that factual storytellers (that is, historians) are willing to argue about the possible consequences of the stories they tell. But their arguments are built on speculations. And fictional storytellers rarely even *think* about the consequences of their stories. (Consider the fact that William Shakespeare died believing that his titanic stories and their consequences would pretty much die with him.) And if truth be told, historians treat their factual stories rather like fictions, especially if they are colossal stories. They make windy declarations about a colossal event's possible consequences...and then they saunter off to another colloquium. But we who have invested our emotions, and even our lives, in the story of that colossal event, we yearn to derive a sense of *meaning* from it. And the greater the story, the greater our yearning.

We shouldn't blame historians for dancing around the possible consequences from their colossal histories. We've seen how hard it is just to *recount* the story of a global pandemic, or simply one of its "consensual narratives." Amplifying that narrative's melody into a symphony of meaningful echoes is enough to boggle the brain. Hence the aforementioned headache. So what we're going to do in this chapter is see whether we can use the lens of *metaphor* to discern some meaningful consequences in the stories of the global pandemics we have encountered. And in the final chapter, we will seek the meaningful consequences that are likely to arise from the coronavirus pandemic, although its actual outcomes are greatly obscured by the fog of the future.

It's a daunting prospect, isn't it? But let's be clear. The task of deriving meaning from a large and unruly event is *always* a daunting prospect. Same applies to deriving meaning from a large story that would seem much less complex...like a great play. In truth, identifying precise consequences of meaning from *any* large story—factual or fictional—is impossible. It's more of an art than a science. But that doesn't mean that it's not worth attempting. To repeat Alfred Crosby's wise observation, the one with which I began this book—"The big questions are really the only ones worth considering, and colossal nerve has always been a prerequisite for such consideration." So, let's see how far colossal nerve will take us in our attempt to derive a sense of meaning from the maelstrom of consequences that have proceeded from our colossal pandemic stories.

♦ ♦ ♦

On the one hand, it's quite tempting to make glib pronouncements about the causal links between a historic event and the events that follow it.

After all, time marches in a linear direction, right? So some things must necessarily follow other things, and it's very seductive to conclude that the later things were caused by the earlier things. The danger in this tactic becomes clear when we consider the following rules in the game of historical analysis:

1. Just because one thing happens after another thing, that doesn't mean the first thing *caused* the second thing. I may get up before dawn to watch the sun rise, but the sun will still rise, even if I don't get up to watch it. More precisely, rats infested the world's cities *long* before the Black Death. They didn't *cause* the pandemic, they only abetted it.
2. Sometimes one event *will* lead to another event, but not for a very long time, and not in a nearby place. Historians have concluded that the eruption of the Ilopango volcano in El Salvador definitely contributed to the ignition of the Black Death on the Eurasian continent. But that effect occurred several years later and half a world away. Cause and effect can have very elusive relationships in historical time and space.
3. An event like a global pandemic consists of countless details, and its effects are even more numerous than its details. Tying any single detail to any single effect is as impossible as saying which African rodent was the first to transmit plague to a human 10,000 years ago. For one thing, the transmission involved more than one little critter and probably more than one species. What's more, 10,000 years is a laughable estimate that has been rounded off to the nearest millennium for the sake of convenience. So we're back to that headache.
4. The lenses through which we view the events of history are distorted by our contemporary perspective and our personal biases. When we look at historical events and their possible effects, we are forced to analyze circumstances and people so far removed from us that our conclusions are closer to a reading of tea leaves than a scientific analysis. In addition, the historical records are usually sparse and spotty, and they themselves are often distorted lenses into their own time periods.

But before we become completely disheartened, let's remember these three encouraging points:

1. The laws by which Nature governs the world, including its human inhabitants, are relatively consistent. So we can generally rely on Nature's consistency when we're comparing events across time. Gravity has always pulled down, not up, and human beings have always behaved in much the same ways when faced with the monster of pandemic disease.
2. Most historical chroniclers, especially during a pandemic, lacked the means or motivation to completely fabricate their histories. If they had distorted their accounts so far from the facts that they bore no resemblance to what actually happened, no one would have believed or preserved their stories. So the historical records always contain some key kernels of truth.
3. With distance comes perspective, and that holds true for distances in time as well as space. Because we can view the four historic pandemics from distances of centuries, we possess masses of historical and scientific knowledge that were unavailable to the people who lived through those pandemics. For example, we know, as Procopius and John Ronewyk did not, that their worlds were *not* coming to a literal end, and we know that it was a bacillus, and not an angry God, that was causing all the trouble. By contrast, we know that the Aztec nation *was* ending, but we also know the Aztec descendants would preserve an essence of its soul. Greater knowledge bestows greater perspective and insight...and those two things allow us to derive a sense of meaning.

Thus, our search for the meaningful consequences from our global pandemics is aided by historical perspective, abundant knowledge, and the consistency of Nature in its governance of the world and its inhabitants. But most of all, our inquiry gains momentum from our human urge to *seek meaning*, especially in the midst of our most dismal circumstances. Our hunger for meaning is a crucial factor in our quest because we are *not* really seeking the pandemics' factual consequences. What we *mostly* want to know is how these pandemics have changed *us*—as individuals, as societies, and as a species.

Consider the fact that the most important rituals conducted by the ancient Greeks were the Eleusinian mysteries—ancient rites organized around a fearsome underground descent that was designed to ignite an encounter between the initiates and their personal sense of meaning. The Eleusinian mysteries were practiced for more than two thousand years, and their general structure is well known to modern scholars. But the specific contents of the Eleusinian rituals remain a mystery to this day.

Now, we know that human beings are *terrible* at keeping secrets, so we must assume that the Eleusinian initiates kept their rituals secret because the things they experienced in their descents to the sacred cave were too personal and too potent to be expressed. What each person encountered in that terrifying darkness was an enlightenment beyond words, a priceless illumination for which the initiate paid dearly with humility and surrender.

The meaningful consequences that we seek from our encounters with Pestilence are likely to be an Eleusinian kind of illumination—less about historical facts and statistical deductions, and more about the precious gems of consciousness that are ignited by immense suffering, courage, and humility. So let's make one final descent into the worlds of our deadliest pandemics, and see if we can mine some jewels of enlightenment out of all that darkness.

Meaningful Consequences from the Plague of Justinian

For want of a nail the shoe was lost.
For want of a shoe the horse was lost.
For want of a horse the rider was lost.
For want of a rider the message was lost.
For want of a message the battle was lost.
For want of a battle the kingdom was lost.
And all for the want of a horseshoe nail.

– Medieval proverb of unknown origin

When most people study a global pandemic, the first thing they ask is how many people it killed. This is a reasonable question, because we assume that a body count is the most meaningful statistic in any deadly event. We also assume that it is the easiest statistic to obtain.

Neither assumption is true.

In fact, it is impossible to ascertain the exact number of people who have died in any pandemic. That is not simply a problem with the archaic systems of recordkeeping that were employed in the past, especially during pandemic chaos. Even during modern periods of relative health, experts estimate that a variety of factors—logistic, financial, religious, political, and emotional—make the reported number of human deaths far less than the actual number.[117] And this has been especially true during the coronavirus pandemic.[118] It is estimated that its current death toll in 2022 is over 15 million people, more than double the previous count.[119] Historians debate the accuracy of all statistics, but the perennial inaccuracy of mortality records suggests that when it comes to counting dead people, the historical canvas should be painted with very cautious brush strokes.

This argument is particularly important when we examine the consequences of the Plague of Justinian. Earlier I mentioned an article that appeared in December 2019 and made *big* news...in the world of academic historians. (Which is probably why you missed it. Don't feel bad. I missed it, too.) The article was controversial because its authors proposed that the Plague of Justinian was, to quote their bold title, "inconsequential."[120]

Now, as you might imagine, labeling our first recorded global pandemic as "inconsequential" is the historian's version of dropping the mic. The authors of this provocative piece describe their extensive review of post-Justinian documents, from which they sought evidence of pandemic-induced changes in populations, harvest reports, political stability, and financial fluctuation. In the end, the authors of the article conclude that, based on the uneven patterns of post-plague data, "the Justinianic plague did not play a significant role in the transformation of the Mediterranean world or Europe."[121] Oh. So not only the world did *not* come to an end from the Plague of Justinian, as Procopius and his colleagues feared it would, these authors conclude that the world barely flinched. Really?

Coincidentally (or not), May 2020 saw the re-publication of another academic article, this time focusing on the effects of the Justinianic Plague in the Middle East.[122] Its authors also combed the financial, historic, and

117. Baskar, Pranav. "Why The Pandemic Could Change The Way We Record Deaths" *NPR/OPB*, September 25, 2020. https://www.npr.org/sections/goatsandsoda/2020/09/25/914073217/why-the-pandemic-could-change-the-way-we-record-deaths

118. "Estimation of total mortality due to Covid-19." *Institute for Health Metrics and Evaluation*, May 6, 2021. https://www.healthdata.org/sites/default/files/files/Projects/COVID/2021/102_briefing_United_States_of_America_17.pdf

119. Nolen, Stephanie and Karan Deep Singh. "India Is Stalling the W.H.O.'s Efforts to Make Global Covid Death Toll Public" *New York Times*, April 16, 2022 https://www.nytimes.com/2022/04/16/health/global-covid-deaths-who-india.html

120. Mordechai, Lee, Merle Eisenberg, Timothy Newfield, Adam Izdebski, Janet Kay, and Hendrik Poinar. "The Justinianic Plague: An inconsequential pandemic?" *Proceedings of the National Academy of Sciences*, December 17, 2019. https://doi.org/10.1073/pnas.1903797116

121. *Ibid.* p. 1

122. Pamuk, Şevket and Maya Shatzmiller. "Plagues, Wages and Economic Change in the Islamic Middle East, 700-1500" *The Journal of Economic History* 196, 2014. Summarized in https://islamiclaw.blog/2020/05/05/economic-impact-and-consequences-of-the-plagues-on-the-medieval-middle-east-2/

cultural evidence for the post-plague period, but they focused on the Middle East, which underwent a period of massive prosperity and development from the 8th to 11th centuries CE—an era often referred to as "The Golden Age of Islam." Although the records cited in this article also report uneven levels of death and decline following the plague, the authors found abundant evidence suggesting that the plague eventually led to a climate of economic freedom and expansion that directly enabled the Islamic world to bloom and flourish.

This expansionist view on the aftermath of the Justinianic Plague is repeated in a variety of other analyses, including in the most comprehensive and accessible book on the subject—William Rosen's *Justinian's Flea.*[123] In his conclusion, Rosen speculates, and quite conservatively, about the consequences of the Plague of Justinian. He first observes, as I have, that no one can claim with assurance that later events are necessarily the consequences of earlier events. However, Rosen feels confident enough to offer this conclusion, based on his voluminous research:

> The most long-lasting effect of the plague was not in its initial impact, but the way in which its aftershocks remade the topography of Europe and the Mediterranean. As the demon washed across the lands once ruled by Rome, it left behind tidal pools: the distinctive regions in which proto-nations like the Franks, Lombards, Saxons, Slavs, and Goths could coalesce and combine into polities called France, Spain, England...and, a few centuries later, into Italy, Germany, and the Netherlands. The consequence [was then] the birth of Europe.[124]

William Rosen and the authors of the article on the consequences of plague in the Islamic world were not fabricating evidence to reach their conclusions that the Plague of Justinian had an enormous effect on its world. And the authors of the "inconsequential" plague article were not ignoring evidence in order to reach their conclusions. So how do we resolve this conundrum in our search for some consequential impact from humanity's first recorded encounter with global pestilence? If the Justinianic Plague left so little evidence of its lethality, as the "inconsequential" authors conclude, how did it manage to facilitate the birth of Europe and the dawn of Islam's Golden Age?

123. Rosen, William *Justinian's Flea: The First Great Plague and the End of the Roman Empire*. New York: Penguin, 2007.

124. Ibid. p 324.

To reconcile these conflicting opinions, let's return to something we learned from the 50-year silence that followed the 1918 flu pandemic. Specifically, we encountered a fundamental axiom of all historical analysis, which is that, "The absence of evidence can *never* be taken as evidence of absence." The 1918 flu killed upward of 50 million people in less than 18 months and it ended the first global war. But if Alfred Crosby hadn't written his 1976 book, the historians of the future would have reviewed the lack of post-pandemic commentary on the flu and decided that the 1918 pandemic was no more than an "inconsequential" outbreak of war-born disease.

So let's not worry about consequences that can't be found, and look instead at the inarguable consequences that can't be denied. Let's consider the fact, disputed by *no* one, that one thing this plague *did* do was to shatter Justinian's dream of a reunited Roman Empire. Justinian conquered and consolidated much of the territory that had been Rome's. But his vision was annihilated by years of bad climate, widespread famine, and prolonged war, topped by the cataclysm of a plague that struck with lethal ferocity in the population centers of Justinian's empire (including his capitol of Constantinople). Two decades after Justinian's death, his reconstituted empire collapsed.

The question is, *how* did it collapse? Well, the Roman Empire employed a very centralized system of governance, in both its original form and in Justinian's. Some authority was granted to regional leaders, but when it came to the important elements of governance, "all roads led to Rome" (even when Justinian's "Rome" was Constantinople). This fact is crucial to the puzzle because the control centers for Justinian's empire were also its most densely populated places, and we know that plague is most lethal in places where humans (along with rats and fleas) are most densely populated. There were fewer of those densely populated places in the 6th century than in the 14th, so it was inevitable that the plague would kill fewer people in the 6th century than the 14th. But the key point is that even though proportionately fewer people died in the Justinianic Plague than in the Black Death, *the people who died in the Plague of Justinian comprised most of the people who ran Justinian's world.* Their loss wasn't immediately noticeable; it was more like that "symphony of echoes," followed by a vast and ominous silence.

In a perfect world, all individuals are of equal value in the eyes of Nature (or whomever). But when it comes to a society whose power and control are highly centralized, the people who live and work in the densely populated hubs of power (plague-infested during a plague pandemic) will undoubtedly be the people who wield more "consequential" influence than the people who live in the sparsely populated (and therefore plague-protected) hinterlands. In a centralized government, "hub" dwellers maintain the social order and preserve a functioning society. When they die, the system dies. In other words, it wasn't how *many* people died in Justinian's plague that made the difference in what came later. Rather, it was *which* people died that made for the consequences that endure to the present day. All that was needed was a focused die-off in the empire's command centers of governance, travel, and commerce, and that ensured that the entire empire would be crippled. And soon thereafter, the empire died.

To get a sense of how extensive these effects were, here is the First Roman Empire in 117 CE:

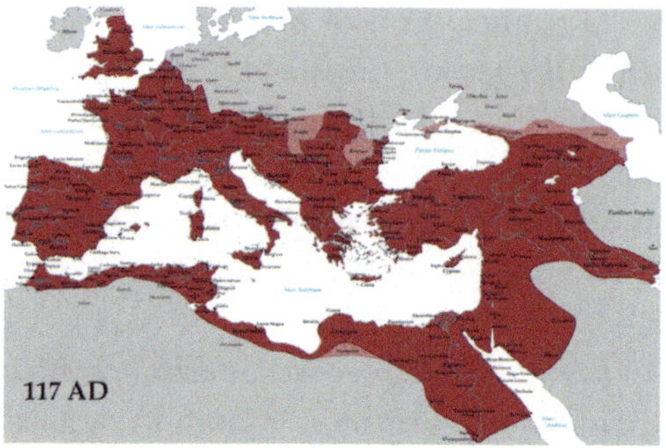

And here is Justinian's Second Roman Empire, not long after the plague stuck (circa 555 CE):

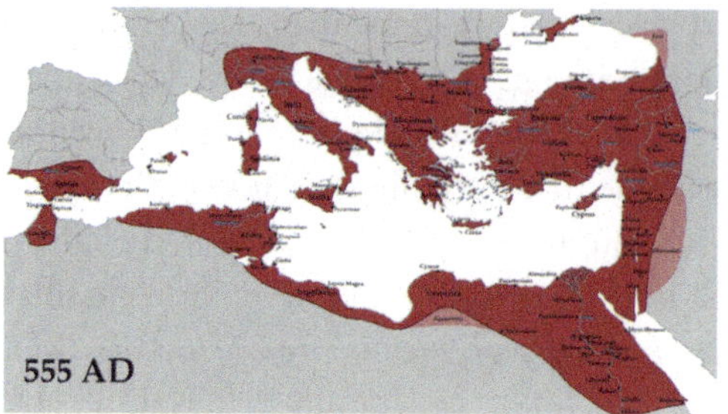

And here is approximately how things looked politically from the 6th to the 11th century CE...which historians now call "the early Middle Ages," but which most of us know as "the Dark Ages" (All images from Wikimedia):

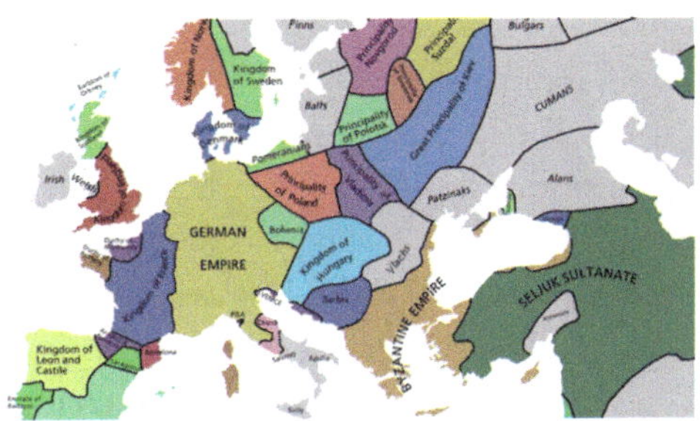

Each of those little blobs of color (aside from the Islamic caliphate in the east) were proto-nations that spent *500 years* feuding among themselves. That means that for the same amount of time that has passed between Columbus's landing in the New World and your bowl of Corn Flakes this morning, all of Europe and much of the Mediterranean floundered in turmoil among a rabble of micro-communities. These fiefdoms were in perpetual conflict, and subject to only brief periods of slight oversight. During this 500-year period, most trade, travel, and law were perilously chaotic, and the shreds of Greco-Roman culture languished inside monasteries.

In other words, for the half-millennium after the collapse of the Second Roman Empire, life in Europe was *calamitous*, to borrow Barbara Tuchman's chilling adjective. The collapse didn't happen in a moment or month. But its effect must have seemed endless to those who suffered through those 500 years, even though they couldn't understand its cause. The Roman systems of order collapsed within the relatively short space of a few decades following the Justinianic plague. Life descended to levels of danger, uncertainty, and hardship that those formerly Roman lands hadn't known for centuries. The world of Islam recovered more quickly than that of Europe, but even there, it took *centuries* for the "Golden Age" to emerge. Simply put, life around the Mediterranean and into the Middle East became torturous after the Plague of Justinian. It is no longer academically acceptable to refer to this era as "the Dark Ages," but even the kindest review of its conditions makes clear why that label came into common use.

You don't have to die in a pandemic in order to feel as if your life has been ended by it. You don't have to volunteer for an initiation into the mysteries of the underworld gods in order to be dragged down to their depths and painfully transformed by them. Sometimes—maybe most times—you're abducted without notice or consent, and your former life is abruptly terminated.

Abduction into a traumatic transformation is, in fact, the storyline of the myth upon which the Eleusinian mysteries were founded. They were derived from a prehistoric tale about a *kore* or "nameless maiden"—later called Persephone by the Greeks—who was sheltered and pampered by her mother-goddess, whom the Greeks called Demeter. The maiden was perfectly content...until the day when she was picking flowers in a meadow and the ground cracked open beneath her feet. Up from the crevasse sprang a black team of horses pulling a black chariot, driven by a charioteer clothed entirely in black. The driver grabbed Persephone, swung the chariot around, and then drove the whole affair back into the black earth...which promptly slammed shut behind him.

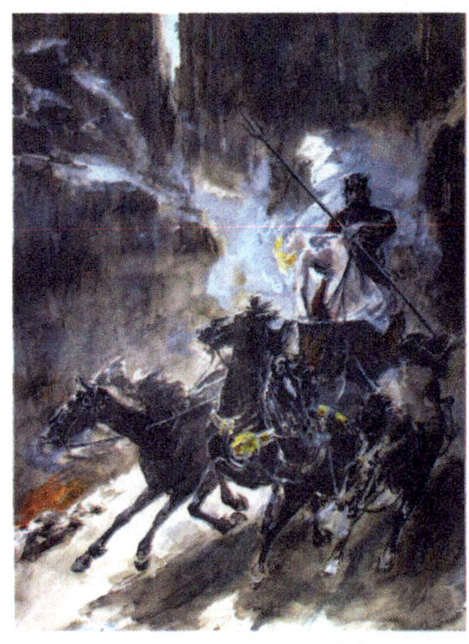

The Abduction of Persephone (1888)
Ulpiano Checa (Wikimedia)

The charioteer was Hades, the god of an underworld that was also called Hades, which was a place in Greek mythology that held both fearsome darkness and immense riches. Hades wanted a wife, so he abducted Persephone. And there she lay, languishing upon his subterranean couch, while her mother wailed and stormed on the Earth above. It was only when Demeter threatened to starve all the human worshippers of the Olympian gods (she was the goddess who controlled the harvests) that Zeus relented and ordered Hades to return Persephone to the upper world.

Now here's where the story gets really interesting... Persephone knew that if she ate anything in Hades, she would be compelled by the laws of Nature to return there every year. So before she left, she ate six seeds of a pomegranate, ensuring that she would be obliged to spend six months of each year in the underworld. Thus, spring and summer became the months when Persephone lives in the upper world with her mother, while everything blooms and gives harvest. And in fall and winter, she returns to reign in an underworld of rich inner darkness with her husband Hades.

In all of Greek mythology, Persephone is the only deity who undergoes such a profound transformation, and she is the only deity who can dwell in both the upper and lower worlds. For these reasons, Persephone and her story came to symbolize any deep and drastic descent that forces us to grow in ways we never would grow otherwise. Persephone regained and enjoyed the pleasures of her pastoral upbringing, but she held tightly to the wisdom and riches that she acquired during her time in the underworld. Indeed, she became the Queen of Hades.

Such painful abductions into consciousness are life-changing and they can even be life-saving. But they are *never* easy. Well, what profound transformation could possibly be easy? The caterpillar must liquify itself in order to become a butterfly—which is why it became another symbol for transformation for the ancient Greeks.

The authors of the 2019 article on the Plague of Justinian concluded that just because its death counts weren't as large as Procopius claimed, the Justinian plague was itself "inconsequential." But our journey through pandemic history has taught us that those who physically survive a pestilence can still die—they just die in a different way. Pandemic survivors find their lives and their worlds so utterly changed by the pestilence that they might as well have been killed by it. Those who escape literal death during a pandemic usually find themselves re-entering a world that is profoundly different from the one they inhabited before the contagion burst into flame. And they often find that they themselves have been so profoundly changed that they are different people from the people they were before the pandemic began.

If there are meaningful consequences from the Plague of Justinian, this could well be one of them. Since the fall of Justinian's empire, Western culture has occasionally returned to imperial servitude—under the cross of the Roman Church, under the banner of the British Empire, under the Soviet sickle, under the Nazi boot. But the spirit of independent nationalism that was born in the wake of the Justinianic Plague—with all its feuding and chaos—has burned itself into the human psyche. And that spirit has resisted all permanent regressions to lock-step totalitarianism.

There may be no solid proof that Justinian's plague was as deadly as Procopius claimed, nor that it gave birth to an independent, multinational consciousness by releasing Europe and the Middle East from the iron grip of the Roman imperial system. But as you have seen, these colossal pandemic events must be considered from a colossal distance (which, yes, does require colossal nerve). Considered from this vast distance of time and space, it is hard to find another event, aside from the Plague of Justinian, that could have precipitated the colossal changes in social consciousness that took place during that same time period. If the loss of a nail from the shoe of a horse can precipitate the loss of a kingdom, what might be lost (and later gained) when an entire Pestilential Horseman shatters the campaign of an aspiring tyrant to resurrect the Roman Empire?

Meaningful Consequences from the Black Death

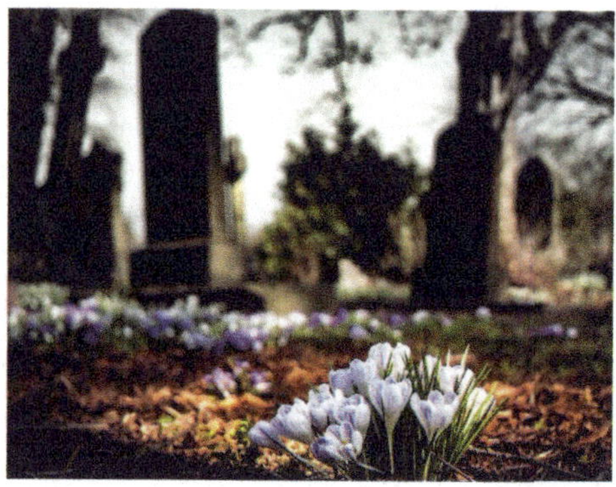

(Wikimedia)

To sue to live, I find I seek to die;
And, seeking death, find life: let it come on.
– William Shakespeare, *Measure for Measure,* **III.i**

There's a certain sense of freedom
in a total loss of hope.
You can miss a lot when you tie a knot
in the end of every rope.
– Cosy Sheridan[125]

Historians may debate the deadly consequences of the Plague of Justinian, but no historian has had the audacity to suggest that the Black Death was anything less than disastrous for humanity. The rates of mortality varied across the map, as they do in any pandemic, and the death counts were even

125. Sheridan, Cosy. "Demeter's Lost Daughter" *The Pomegranate Seed,* Amazon Music, © 2004. Used by the gracious permission of Cosy Sheridan. (https://cosysheridan.com/) (https://www.amazon.com/Pomegranate-Seed-Cosy-Sheridan/dp/B000QR0YLM)

more uncertain during this viral catastrophe than they were during the rest of the Middle Ages. But all historians agree that more than a third of the world's population died between 1347 and 1353. And in many parts of the world, it was reliably documented that over half the population died—in some places within the space of a single year.

In Europe, the worst of the pandemic lasted for the first five years, and the most appalling levels of mortality occurred during the first two years. In the Italian city of Florence, for example, it is certain that at least 60% of the people died within two years, and subsequent waves of the plague prevented Florence's population from returning to its pre-plague level for nearly two hundred years. Today, we talk about experiencing "pandemic burnout" after two years in the grip of the novel coronavirus. In 2022, it has killed approximately 15 million people who represent 0.19% of the current population. Now, imagine that *nearly two billion* people had died in these past two years...130 people dead of plague for every one coronavirus victim. That is *at least* the proportion of pandemic death that most people in the 14th century had experienced by 1353.

And it wasn't finished after the first five years. The fires of the Black Death blazed back and forth across Europe for *400 years*. The hot coals of its contagion seethed continually throughout those four centuries, but its most noteworthy conflagrations occurred during 1360–63, 1374, 1400, 1438–39, 1456–57, 1464–66, 1481–85, 1500–03, 1518–31, 1544–48, 1563–66, 1573–88, 1596–99, 1602–11, 1623–40, 1644–54, and 1664–67. Moreover, those numbers don't begin to address its incinerating outbreaks in places like Asia and Africa, where death records were maintained much more sporadically or else were lost altogether. And it hardly needs to be said that no statistic can begin to touch the *emotional* experience of this catastrophe. Here is one account of what this pandemic *felt* like:

Father abandoned child, wife husband, one brother another;
for this illness seemed to strike through the breath and sight.
And so they died.

And none could be found to bury the dead for money or friendship.
Members of a household brought their dead to a ditch
as best they could, without priest, without divine offices ...
great pits were dug and piled deep with the multitude of dead.
And they died by the hundreds both day and night ...
And as soon as those ditches were filled more were dug ...

And I, Agnolo di Tura ... buried my five children with my own hands.
And there were also those who were so sparsely covered with earth
that the dogs dragged them forth and
devoured many bodies throughout the city.

There was no one who wept for any death,
for all awaited death.

And so many died that all believed it was the end of the world.
– Agnolo di Tura, Chronicler in Siena, Italy, 1348[126]

There is a point past which a large volume of death can render us incapable of feeling—by which I mean we become incapable of feeling *anything*. We become numb, devoid of *all* feeling—"as hollow and empty as the spaces between stars."[127] This void state is what is meant by the saying that "A single death is a tragedy; a million deaths is a statistic."[128] In other words, at the moment we receive a report of death—by the ones or the one millions—we respond in reverse proportion to the lethal head count. The more dead people, the less we are able to feel.

But in the long run, those dead millions burn an indelible brand into our hearts. Few of us can remain numb forever. And over time, the absence of those dead millions burns another kind of brand into us—into our unconscious minds, into our collective hearts, and into our world.

This, it seems, is what happened during the first and worst years of the Black Death, and then during its four centuries of afterburn. There was an initial period in which, "There was no one who wept for any death, for all awaited death," as poor Agnolo Di Tura wrote in 1348. And there was a second period in which people trudged as best they could through what remained of life. But when the people of Europe awakened from their benumbed nightmare, somewhere in the late 1350s, they found themselves in a very different world from the one out of which they had been abducted ten years earlier. And even more different were the worlds of 1460, 1560, 1660, and 1760, and during the following 400 years of eruptions by "the Great Mortality."

126. Rogers, P.M. *Aspects of Western Civilization.* New York: Prentice Hall, 2000, pp 353–65.

127. Chandler, Raymond. *The Long Goodbye.* New York: Vintage Crime/Black Lizard, 2002, p 252.

128. Author unknown, though usually credited (erroneously) to Joseph Stalin, who did cite it, and whose certainly manifested its spirit through the mass murders committed by his regime.

The pre-plague world of 1346 had functioned quite strictly, according to the social order that had accrued during the previous eight centuries after Justinian's empire collapsed. Post-Justinian societies (especially in Europe but also in other parts of the world) had become rigidly structured and stratified. In Europe, people were born into the classes of nobility, clergy, warrior, or laborer...or else they barely existed in the eyes of the social order. And the distance between a member of the nobility and a farm laborer (also called a *serf*) was equivalent to the spaces between the stars. There also existed some migrating peoples—those who practiced medicine, the trades, or the arts. But the formal practices of such professions, which were not sanctioned by the Church, were restricted to outcast groups such as the Jews, the Cathars, and the Muslims.

The belief systems of the Early Middle Ages were as highly structured as the societies that practiced them. Indeed, the prevailing belief system in Europe—Roman Catholicism—served as the fundamental rule of European life during the centuries leading up to the Black Death. During these centuries, the Roman Church exerted a control so increasingly pervasive that, by the 13th century, it was difficult for most Europeans to conceive of a reality outside of the one dictated by the Church.

To be sure, there were small but crucial sparks of impending change in pre-plague Europe. For example, in 1320—twenty-seven years before the European outbreak of the Black Death—the poet/statesman Dante Alighieri published *The Divine Comedy*, a long narrative poem that is now considered one of the iconic works of world literature. Dante's journey begins with a descent into the *Inferno*—the first of three "cantiche" (songs) that continue into the *Purgatorio*, and end in the *Paradiso*. Although *The Divine Comedy* was ostensibly a description of the afterlife as the early medievals saw it, it actually depicted key elements of *all* reality, practical and spiritual, as they were construed in the Middle Ages. And because the poems were written in allegorical form, Dante was able to include materials from the Islamic and Greco-Roman cultures that were technically forbidden by the Roman Church.

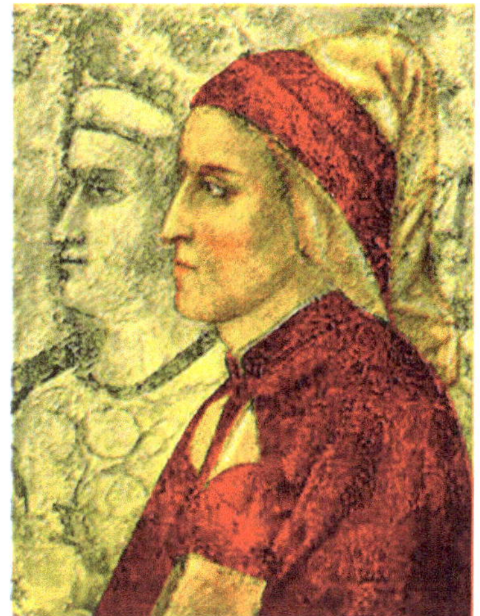

Dante Aligheiri (1300 CE) Barghello Palace, Florence (Wikimedia)

The Divine Comedy shows that the seeds of cultural evolution, and cultural *revolution*, were already germinating in the soil of the medieval unconscious. More compelling and more pertinent to our quest is the fact that Dante's journey into the afterlife begins in a way that is very similar to Persephone's descent to her transformative experience in Hades. Take a look at these introductory lines to Dante's epic tale:

> Midway in our life's journey, I went astray
> From the straight road and woke to find myself
> Alone in a dark wood. How shall I say
>
> what wood that was! I never saw so drear,
> so rank, so arduous a wilderness!
> Its very memory gives a shape to fear
>
> Death could scarce be more bitter than that place!
> But since it came to good, I will recount
> all that I found revealed there by God's grace.
>
> How I came to it I cannot rightly say,
> so drugged and loose with sleep had I become
> when I first wandered there from the True Way...
>
> Just as a swimmer, who with his last breath
> flounders ashore from the perilous seas, might turn
> to memorize the wise water of his death—
>
> So did I turn, my soul still fugitive
> from death's surviving image, to stare down
> that pass that none had ever left alive.[129]

In other words, Dante is abducted from his reverie to a place of profound darkness beyond mortal existence—"the undiscovered country from whose bourn no traveler returns," as Shakespeare would have Hamlet describe it some 250 years later. This was an abduction into the realm of descending death,

129. From THE DIVINE COMEDY by Dante Alighieri (1327), translated by John Ciardi. Copyright 1954, 1957, 1959, 1960, 1961, 1965, 1967, 1970 by the Ciardi Family Publishing Trust. Used by permission of W. W. Norton & Company. Inc.

and later into a new form of life that lies beyond death. It is a pilgrimage that lasts about six days in Dante's mythic tale. But in the real world, especially the European world, this descent into bottomless demise, followed by a torturous purgatory in a plague-ravaged world, and finally a return into the relative paradise of post-plague life, lasted more than four centuries after the eruption of the Black Death.

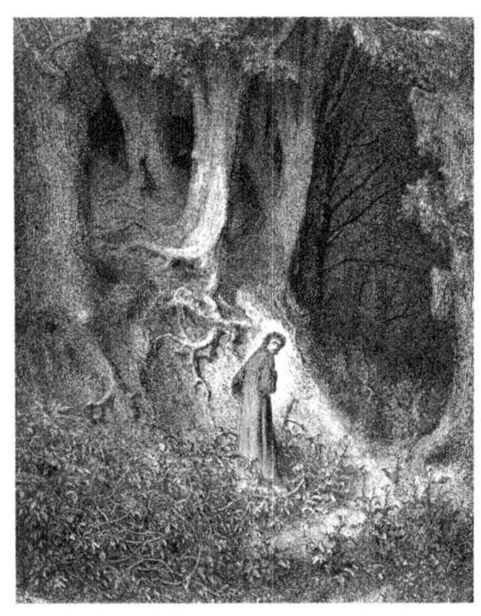

Gustave Doré, *Dante's Inferno, Plate I (1857)* (Wikimedia)

An ocean of words has been written about the aftermath of the Black Death, but *none* of those words have defined it as "inconsequential." (Apparently, there are limits to the audacity of ambitious historians.) Historians may disagree about the nuances of this pandemic's consequences for subsequent generations, but they all seem to agree that the Black Death led to 1) the end of the feudal social system, 2) the birth of what we would now call the "middle class," 3) a rise in the legal and social status of women, and 4) a broad expansion of European consciousness that resulted in the Renaissance. The wisdom of Greco-Roman culture was retrieved from the monasteries, Islamic knowledge was integrated into Western schools of thought, and European culture blossomed and bore fruit in every conceivable discipline.

But the fundamental change that drove it all was a profound transformation in the relationship between European humans and the entity that they called God.

Prior to the Black Death, European faith in God and His Roman Church was nearly absolute. There were marginalized groups that held non-Catholic beliefs—including the Jews, the Muslims, and the Cathars. But those groups were tolerated at best, persecuted in the main, and slaughtered when things got really out of hand. The Catholic God was in charge of everything, and the Catholic Church was His engine of governance.

And then *yersinia pestis* set fire to the medieval world.

In the beginning, the Christian faithful turned to their God and His Church, expecting that both would bless and protect them from the bacterial firestorm. No such luck. The faithful died as fast as the heathen did. And in the case of the Catholic priests and nuns, the devout died even faster than the sinners, because the religious professionals ministered to the sick during the day and returned to their crowded, cloistered communities at night. They died like flies.

The longer the plague continued, and the wider it swung its lethal scythe, the more obvious it became to the medieval Europeans that their God was not wielding the kind of power that the Church had advertised for centuries. Theirs was disillusionment and despair on an epic scale.

Not all was lost. No matter how long or devoutly we human beings have prayed to our more abstract gods, we have always been obliged in the end to kneel before the laws of Nature. And Nature has a way of persevering through the deadliest disasters. The devastating Chernobyl nuclear accident, for example, produced horrible mutations in its immediate wake, but its radiation did not, astonishingly, lead to transgenerational mutations or diseases.[130] Wild crocuses bloom and glow in its dismal cemeteries.

Similarly, the Black Death survivors show emotional trauma in the early plague years, when their art suggests that Death became their new God:

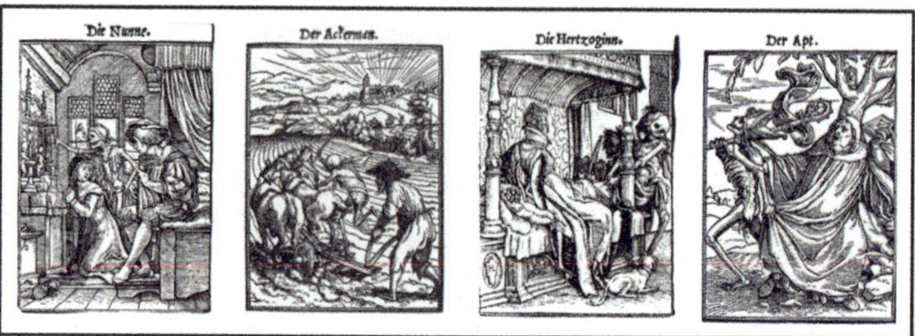

The Dance of Death (Nun, Plowman, Duchess, and *Abbot)* Hans Holbein (1348) (Wikimedia)

But the art of subsequent decades reveals a progressive blossoming of naturalism, humanism, and vitality...

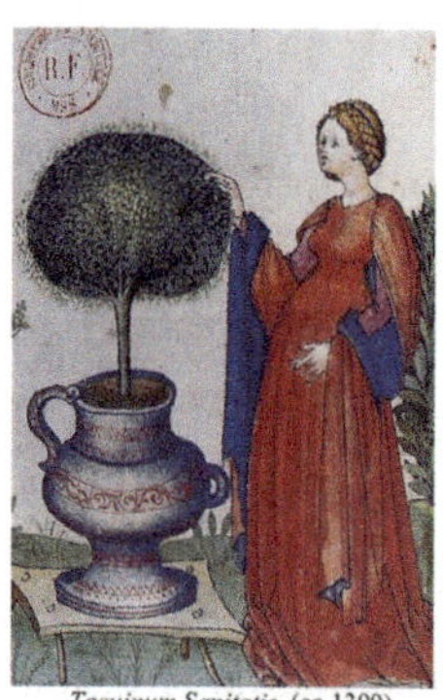

Tacuinum Sanitatis, (ca 1390) (Wikimedia)

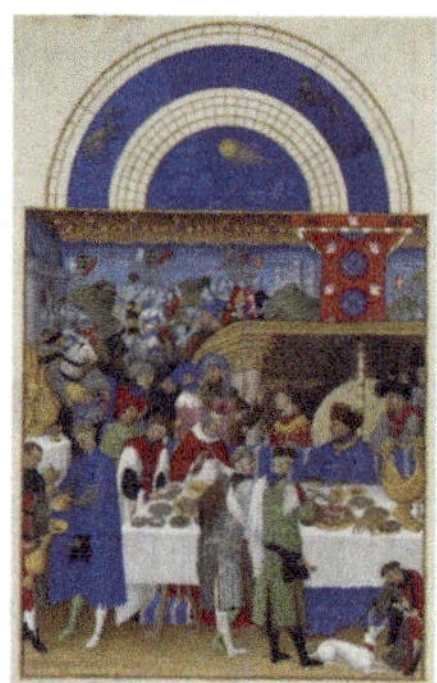

Trés Riches Heures (1420) Limbourg (Wikimedia)

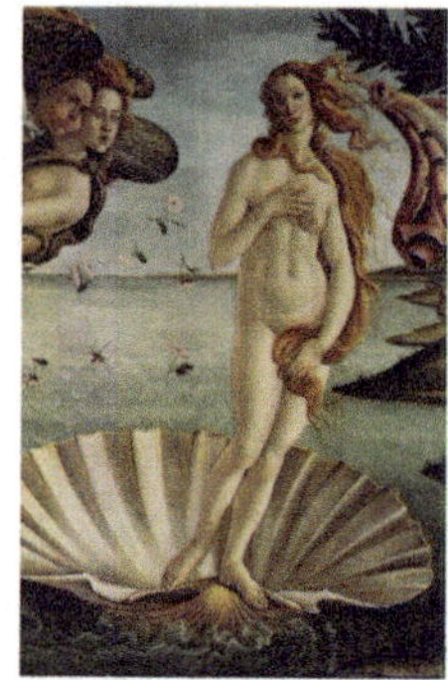

Birth of Venus detail (1485) Botticelli (Wikimedia)

130. "Lack of transgenerational effects of ionizing radiation exposure from the Chernobyl accident." Yaeger, Meredith, Mitchell J. Machiela, Prachi Kothiyal, Michael Dean et al. *Science*, April 22, 2021. https://www.science.org/doi/10.1126/science.abg2365

In the simplest terms, it could be said that the Black Death initially ignited a firestorm of misery and mortality, and quickly thereafter, a massive crisis of faith in God. Had the Devil sent the plague? If so, why didn't God have sufficient power to save humanity from the Devil's mayhem? Or did *God* send the plague? If He did, was it a punishment for humanity's sins? And if it was, what grievous sins had been committed by the people of 1347 that no one had committed before to incite such devastating punishment? And why did the punishment last so long, if the worst of the terrible sinners died off in the first few years of the pestilence? And why did the most pious people, like priests and nuns, seem to die even faster than irreverent persons?

No one had easy answers for these disturbing questions—not during the early years of the Black Death, nor during the decades that followed its devastating combustion. But the light of the human spirit is rarely extinguished by a lack of easy answers. Quite the contrary. An absence of easy answers seems to enhance our human determination to find *other* answers—the not-so-easy answers that are buried in faraway times and forbidden places.

What the survivors of the Black Death found in their search for the not-so-easy answers was the accumulated wisdom in the ancient and contemporary cultures of Greece, Rome, Egypt, Islam, and the Far East. The adamant hand of Roman Catholic orthodoxy would never again hold Europe in its iron grasp. There would still be a Church, but there would also be other forms of Christianity, such as Protestantism, and there would also be increasing numbers of non-Christian believers who would prevent the Church from reasserting its former power.

The decline of Catholic orthodoxy also made possible the rise of a spiritual and practical defiance among the people who lived in the centuries following the Black Death. These were the centuries during which people stopped considering one's physical life as a heathen way-station before one's exalted spiritual afterlife. These were the centuries when most Europeans valued the world of embodied sensation more than the realm of disembodied spirit. The post-plague Europeans turned away from the orthodoxy, asceticism, and obedience that the Roman Church had demanded from the pre-plague Europeans. They embraced instead the values of humanism, individualism, skepticism, diversity, and classical education. It was a revolution on every level of human consciousness.

Building on this philosophical revolution, post-plague Europeans elevated Science as a new regent of reality, and they embraced the scientific practices of measurement, analysis, deduction, and innovation as the instruments of its ministry. Specifically, between the years 1300 and 1600, western Europeans developed a passion for measurement and its practical applications—a passion and practice that is a basis for the pre-eminence of Western culture that has extended into the 21st century.[131] What these plague survivors discovered, while their abstract and unknowable God was dwindling in their esteem, was a new god of analysis. This new deity decoded for the post-plague Europeans the mysteries and masteries of the transformed world that greeted them when they returned from their repeated descents into the inferno of plague. Their methods for the worship of this new god were the practices of the scientific method, starting with something that we now call *pantometry*—a Greek word for "the measurement of everything."

Specifically, this is what those plague survivors developed as their ritual of reverence for the naturalistic god of their post-plague world—a replacement for their former obligation of disembodied and unquestioning worship to the adamant and unknowable Catholic God:

> Reduce what you are trying to think about to the minimum required by its definition. Visualize it on paper, or at least in your mind—be it the fluctuation of wool prices or the course of Mars through the heavens. [Then divide it] into equal quanta [degrees of measurement]. Then you can measure it...that is, you can count the quanta. [Now] you possess a quantitative representation of your subject that is...even in its errors and omissions, precise. You can think about it rigorously. You can manipulate it and experiment with it... Visualization and quantification: together they snap the padlock. Reality is fettered, at least tightly enough and for long enough to get some work out of it, and possibly a law of nature or two.[132]

Empowered by this new form of devotion, the post-plague Europeans emerged, Dante-like, from their descents into their plague-induced Infernos. They returned to new worlds where they could use pantometry to devise tactics for harnessing reality to their purposes. These included:

1. Punctuation—the measurement of written language that is essential for the reading of text silently, thereby expanding the useful application of the printing press.

131. I am once again indebted to Alfred W. Crosby for the following discussion, which is fully articulated in his elegant and insightful book, *The Measure of Reality: Quantification and Western Society 1250-1600.* New York: Cambridge University Press, 1997.

132. Ibid., pp. 228-29.

2. Double-entry bookkeeping with Arabic numerals—essential for the management of complex financial enterprises in banking and trade.
3. Measurement of temperature—essential for experimentation and innovation in medicine and the applied sciences.
4. Musical notation—essential for the performance of multi-part musical composition.
5. Rendering of visual perspective on paper—essential for the creation of realism in artistic, architectural, and mechanical drawings and paintings.
6. Maps metered in longitude and latitude, and accommodated to a spherical world and a "spherical" sky above it—essential for global map-making and transoceanic navigation.

Of course, the authorities who remained active in the Roman Church (and they were *not* inconsequential) put up stiff opposition to much of what was being measured and what was being done with those measurements. Galileo was, after all, imprisoned for his "heretical" discoveries that used the astronomical benefits of pantometry. But just as Nature had prevailed over the Church with *yersinia pestis*, so Nature prevailed over these religious objections to pantometry, and offered up an ocean of skills and information.

This, indeed, is the conclusion of *The Measure of Reality*, one of Alfred Crosby's most ambitious books: that the explosion of pantometry is the single factor explaining how the Muslim geographer Masudi could describe 10th century Europeans as "stupid in mind and heavy in speech...thick, gross, and brutish," while a mere 600 years later, Europeans were flexing the socio-scientific muscles that would expand into what Crosby named "ecological imperialism," and what many authors now refer to as "a global cultural domination by the West."

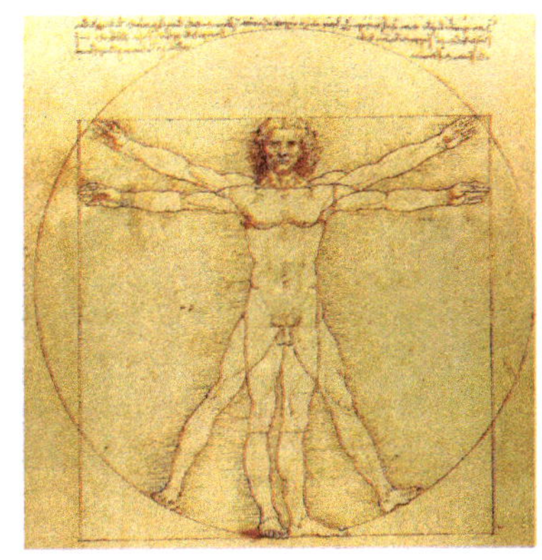

Vitruvian Man (1490 CE) Leonardo da Vinci (Wikimedia)

From 1347 to 1750, Europe was repeatedly abducted into the inferno of *yersinia pestis.* But with each re-emergence into the light, Europeans benefited from whatever one learns in those dark descents, and they put their new consciousness to good use in each of the new worlds that awaited them. One thousand years after the Greek philosopher Protagoras died, we learned that even if he was wrong in saying that "Man is the *measure* of all things," it is very true humankind benefits enormously from being the *measurer* of all things.

The liberation of humanity from the iron yoke of the Roman Church, with its demand for absolute adherence to the laws of a Catholic God, may seem a slight benefit when it is weighed against the conflagration of anguish that erupted during the Black Death. But the scales of justice rarely come into balance, or even relevance, during outbreaks of pandemic disease. After all, the things that are being compared defy any form of measurement, even by the most devout pantometrist. The best we can do is to hold the immeasurable cost of human suffering on one side of our hearts, and the equally incalculable benefits of meaning (such as we find them) on the other side. There can be no balancing of these scales, no reconciling of these accounts. There are only the narratives that remain, and the lives lived and lost, from which we may derive some sense of transformative meaning...hopefully enough meaning that it will redeem the unspeakable misery.

And there is one more important fact to mention about the consequences of the Black Death, a new finding that emphasizes the crucial importance of taking a very long and very careful view with any pandemic story...

On October 19, 2022, *Nature* magazine published a remarkable piece of research conducted by an international team of 31 scientists, led by the bio-geneticist Dr. Luis Barreiro at the University of Chicago.[133] Working in the diverse fields of population biology, social science, and ancient and modern genetics, and using an elegant form of intricate detective work, this team has proven that the human beings who survived the Black Death were largely protected by a particular variant in their DNA. This DNA variant triggered the full-length production of a protein called ERAP2, which prevents plague bacteria from replicating quickly...or at all. This same variant persists in our current human population, and it has presumably granted greater protection against plague to the people who are descended from the Black Death survivors.

Sadly, ERAP2 is also a known risk factor for the autoimmune condition called Crohn's disease. It seems that when an innate immune system can rapidly summon a squad of lethal berserkers to defend the body, it runs the risk that those fierce defenders will later make other mischief with their drive to defend. Then again, better to have an autoimmune disease that impairs one's life, rather than a ghastly pandemic disease that devours it. That being

133. Klunk, Jennifer, Luis B. Barreiro et al. "Evolution of immune genes is associated with the Black Death." *Nature*, October 19, 2022. https://doi.org/10.1038/s41586-022-05349-x

said, this remarkable research has larger implications for the survivors of all future pandemics, though perhaps not for the coronavirus pandemic:

> Will the COVID-19 pandemic have a big impact on human evolution? Barreiro said he doesn't think so because the death rate is so much lower and the majority of people who have died had already had children. In the future, however, he said more deadly pandemics may well continue to shape us at the most basic level. "It's not going to stop. It's going to keep going for sure."[134]

Meaningful Consequences from the Post-Columbian Plural Pandemic

My barn having burned to the ground,
I can now see the moon.
– Mizuta Masahide, 17th century Japanese poet and samurai

Ready must thou be to burn thyself in thine own flame.
How couldst thou become new if thou
have not first become ashes?
– Friedrich Nietzsche, ***Thus Spoke Zarathustra***

Whether we remain the ash or become
the Phoenix is up to us.
– Deng Ming-Dao, Chinese-American philosopher

In terms of destroying bodies and souls, it was the most devastating pandemic in human history. Yes, more people died in the 1918 flu pandemic, and much faster. And the plague pandemics of the 6th and 14th centuries led to the downfall of enormous social and religious structures, as we have

134. Ungar, Laura and The Associated Press. "You might have Crohn's disease, rheumatoid arthritis or lupus because your ancestor survived the Black Death, study says." *Fortune*, October 19, 2022. https://fortune.com/2022/10/19/black-death-bubonic-plague-study-dna-crohns-lupus-arthritis-genes/

seen in the previous two sections. But the plural pandemic of the post-Columbian New World annihilated nearly all of the indigenous people of the northern and southern Americas, and it almost succeeded in eradicating the cultures and traditions of those ancient civilizations. The combination of the conquistadors' brutality, the Inquisition's oppression, the Europeans' exploitation, and a century of relentless pandemics might have obliterated any trace of less resilient peoples.

Somehow, their legacy has survived. Thanks to their ferocity and resilience, the ancient cultures of the pre-Columbian Americas live on, burning brightly to this day in the arts, rituals, fortitude, wisdom, and talents of their descendants. Mind you, it still isn't clear how this miracle came to be. Bernardino documented the soul of the Aztec nation, but even his monumental work went into hiding for two centuries. Human souls and living cultures can't just disappear for two hundred years and still survive. Like a flame that is deprived of air, they simply go *out*. Let's see if we can plumb this miracle for some clues about how the pre-Columbian soul endured.

In the previous sections, we saw a theme of a descent into darkness, followed by a period of disorientation and despair, followed by a return to a new version of the old world, with a challenge to become a new version of oneself—as an individual or a civilization. Persephone's abduction into Hades is echoed in Dante's descent into the Inferno, and their re-entries into life entail the creation of transformed selves that mirror their transformed worlds. These stories are formally called *katabasis* (κατάβασης), which means "go down" in ancient Greek, and they are found everywhere in world mythology—from the earliest Mesopotamian stories, on to Egyptian, Norse, and Greco-Roman myths, farther on to the modern religions of Christianity, Islam, and Hinduism, and even in the sacred lore of Asia, Africa, the Americas, and Pacific Islands. In the Jungian view, the global presence of *katabasis* stories proves that our abduction into a dark underworld, a subterranean chamber where we suffer and are transformed, is a universal element of the human experience.

Sometimes the underworld is a very cold place...as we tend to forget it was in the deepest circle of Dante's Inferno. This is where Dante meets Dis—the dreadful demon whose name means something like "torn asunder" in Greek and Latin. Dis is every energy that dis-members, dis-integrates, dis-tresses, and *dis-eases* the world. Dis and His realm are literally *glacial*—a place where the triple-faced Destroyer floats in an icy lake of blood and guilt while He devours everyone who comes within His grasp.[135] Here is an image of how the medievals depicted Dis and His frozen realm, based on Dante's detailed description:

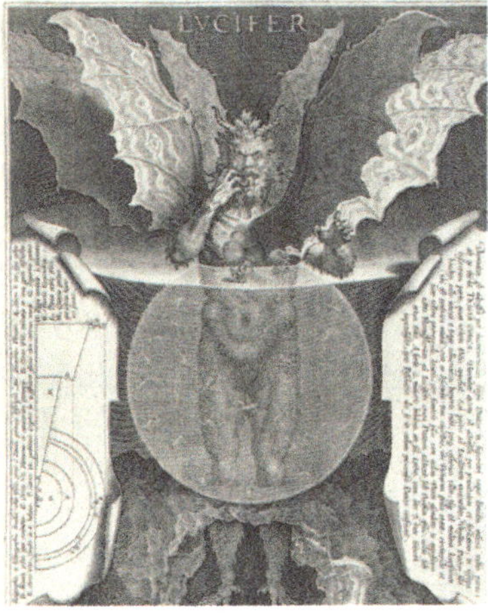

Lucifer, Jan van der Straet (engraving), after Lodovico Cigoli, ca. 1590 CE (Wikimedia)

In versions of the abduction/ descent myth that are more familiar to those of us in Christian and Islamic cultures, the underworld is a place of terrible fire. The Bible's Book of Revelation (21:8) describes the Christian Hell as a "lake that burns with fire and sulfur." The Islamic Hell described in the Quran is called Jahannam and it entails myriad forms of fiery suffering.[136] Abduction into either of these infernal worlds involves blistering anguish.

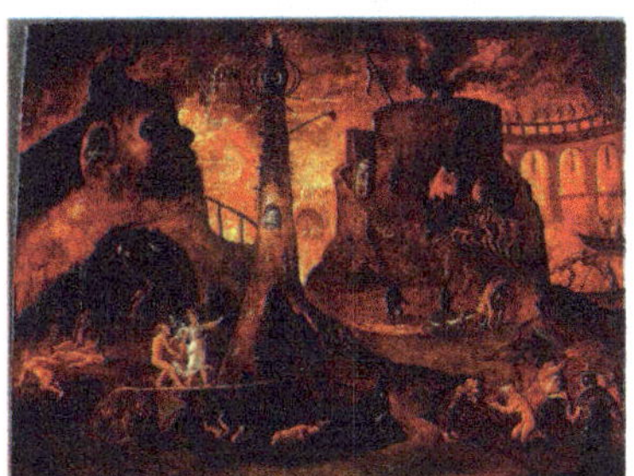

Angel leading souls into Hell (ca. 1490) Student of Hieronymous Bosch (Wikimedia)

In the lore of the world, most people who are taken down to the underworld (usually by death) are destined to remain there forever. Sometimes it is a place of torture, and sometimes it is only a place of non-life. Either way, it is an absolute Ending. But the mythologies of the world also contain—in fact, they *always* contain—stories of mythic persons and entities who descend to the underworld, voluntarily or not, and then return as agents of transformation and evolution. Persephone was one of those persons and Dante

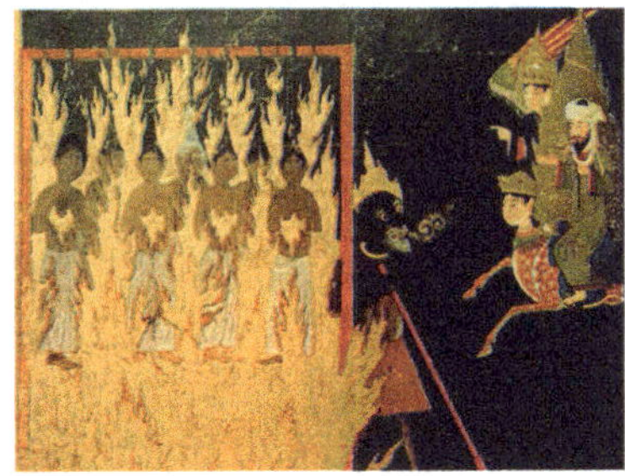

Muhammed visiting Jahannam (ca. 1450) Anonymous artist (Wikimedia)

135. As an interesting corollary to this notion of a frozen lake composed of blood and *guilt*, the teachings of Judaism do not make reference to a specific hell, but rather refer to a state of Gehinnom, a place where souls feel intense *shame* for their misdeeds...although this state can occur during life, as well as after death.

136. https://en.wikipedia.org/wiki/Jahannam

was another. Jesus Christ was one and so was Muhammed.

But there is also a mythic *non*-human creature who is present in nearly *every* mythology of the world, a creature who lives for a fantastically long time, acquiring immense wisdom and power, and who then surrenders to a descent into sacred flames—whether by will or by destiny. These are not flames that merely torture. They are flames that immolate, consuming this creature in a sacrificial fire until nothing is left but cold ash. And then—either immediately or after vast time—the creature or its offspring rises from the ashes, born anew to bring its power and wisdom back to the world.

The name of this creature that is best known to us is *phoenix*, but it has had many other names as it has appeared in the lore of cultures around the world. Here are a few, along with their images:

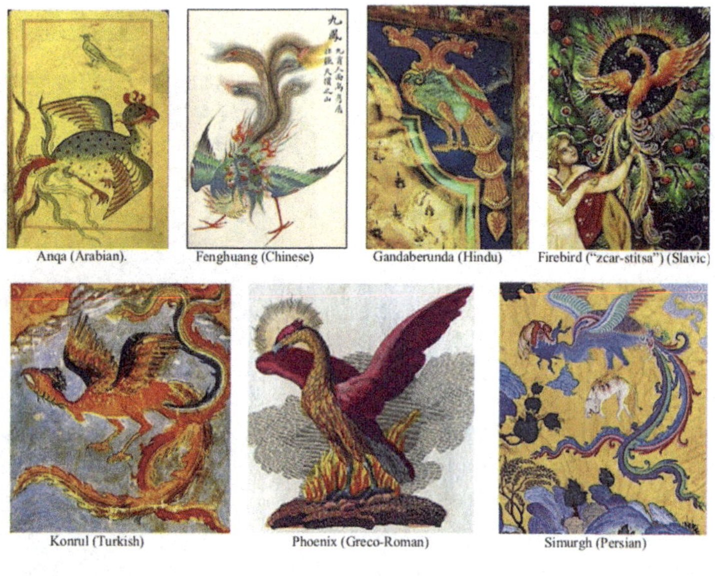

Anqa (Arabian). Fenghuang (Chinese) Gandaberunda (Hindu) Firebird ("zcar-stitsa") (Slavic)

Konrul (Turkish) Phoenix (Greco-Roman) Simurgh (Persian)

(All Wikimedia)

In each of these cultures, this creature is considered miraculous, mysterious, and transformative. But in most cases, the creature is only one of many divine entities. To the Mesoamerican peoples, however, this creature was a primary deity, a giver of life and a bringer of light in the darkest times. His name is *Quetzalcoatl*, but he has also been known as "the Feathered Serpent."

Born of either two gods or a human virgin, Quetzalcoatl makes his first documented appearance around 900 BCE in an Olmec (pre-Aztec) site near the current Mexican state of Tabasco. After that debut, the worship of the

Feathered Serpent spread across the region until Quetzalcoatl had become one of the three most powerful deities in the Mesoamerican pantheon. He is master of the wind, learning, commerce, the arts, the priesthood, and the rising of the sun. And in a more practical moment, Quetzalcoatl brought corn (maize) to feed humankind.

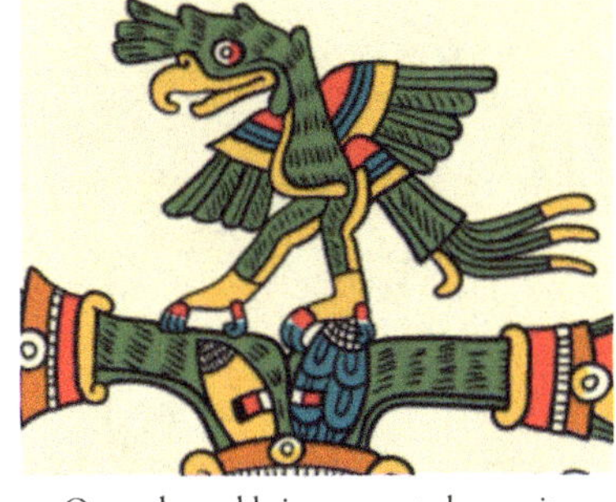

Queztalcoatal brings corn to humanity (Detail) (*Codex Borgia)* (Wikipedia)

The journey of Quetzalcoatl was not without hardship, being marked by two stories of terrible descent and great redemption. In the first, the Feathered Serpent cast himself into a great fire as an act of remorse, and then rose to become the "morning star" (Venus), which was the guide for planting and harvest in Mesoamerica. And in the second story, Quetzalcoatl descended into the Mesoamerican underworld, called Mictlan, after humankind was destroyed by a natural disaster...for the fourth time. From the remnants of those deceased humans, and from the blood of his own body, Quetzalcoatl formed a "humankind of the fifth-world," the humans who greeted Columbus and his successors.

In 2012, the multi-disciplined Mesoamerican scholars Virginia Fields, John Pohl, and Virginia Lyall created an astonishing exhibit entitled "Children of the Plumed Serpent: The Legacy of Quetzalcoatl in Ancient Mexico." Initially designed for the Los Angeles County Museum of Art, the exhibit went on to tour other museums and was eventually published as a book.[137] The research anthology compiled by these scholars documents a powerful alliance of Mesoamerican nations in south-central Mexico that was able to survive the devastating effects of the conquistadors, the Spanish Inquisition, and the plural pandemics, well enough to establish an enduring culture of autonomy and vitality. This was, and is, a multi-nation community of indigenous peoples, centered in the pilgrimage site of Cholula, near Mexico City. It was, and is, a community united by shared social, political and religious values, all of which were, and still are, founded in the worship of Quetzalcoatl. This community's astonishing success is evidenced by the indigenous customs and values that continue to flourish in south-central Mexico, and by the persistent popularity and worship of Quetzalcoatl that continues today,

137. Fields, Virginia, John Pohl, and Virginia Lyall. *Children of the Plumed Serpent: The Legacy of Quetzalcoatl in Ancient Mexico.* Los Angeles, CA: Scala Publishers, 2012.

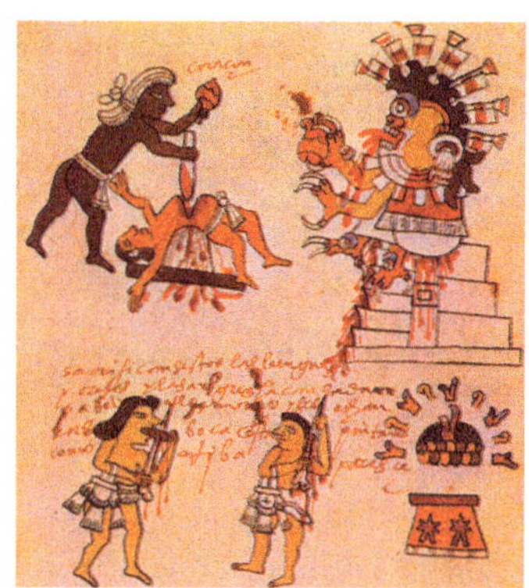

Aztec rituals of human sacrifice and cannibalism (16th century CE) *Codex Tudela* (Wikipedia)

including semi-annual festivals in Cholula dedicated to the Plumed Serpent.

And here is one more important consequence that emerged from that pestilential time in post-Columbian Mesoamerica...

It is a well-documented truth, albeit very painful for our modern selves to acknowledge, that the Mesoamerican peoples anciently included in their sacramental rites the practices of human sacrifice and the ingestion of those sacrificed people. These practices were many centuries old when the conquistadors arrived, and the practices were continued into the century after their arrival, despite ferocious efforts by the Spanish conquerors and the Catholic Inquisition to stop them. But there is *no* record of further human sacrifice, nor of any cannibalism, after 1600, even though Quetzalcoatl was still ardently worshipped in much of central America...as he is to this day. To borrow Alfred Crosby's framing once again, the only factor that can account for this "colossal" change in a culture's ancient practices, especially its death practices, is another "colossal" death factor...like a plural pandemic that annihilates nearly 90% of the population. Rituals of human sacrifice—for any reason, no matter how holy—might well have seemed meaningless, redundant, or at the very least, obsolete, after that pestilential holocaust.

There is no way to resurrect the millions of people who suffered and died in the plural pandemics of the post-Columbian New World. But metaphorically speaking, it seems that the archetypal energy of Quetzalcoatl surrendered to that holocaust of anguish, immolated himself in its flames, and descended into the underworld of Mictlan again in order to create out of the Mesoamerican bloodlines and his own mythic potency a "humankind of the *sixth* world"—a nation of "children of the plumed serpent" who are vibrantly alive and flourishing today.

These tales of multiple humanities may strain our Euro-American ears, but perhaps we should give a bit more credence to the sacred stories that the pre-Columbian peoples were composing from the rich soil of their souls and the prehistoric relics they found in their land. Consider this remarkable creature, whose remnants are located in (at least) what is now northern

Mexico. One of the largest known flying animals of all time, its skeleton has been fully assembled and it has been aptly named...*Quetzalcoatlus northropi*:

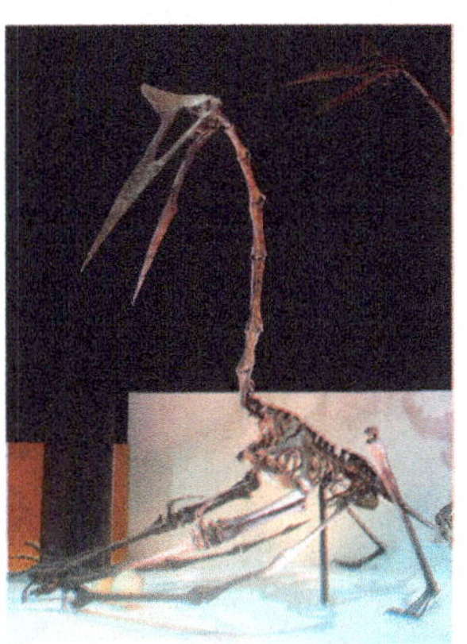

Skeleton of *Quetzalcoatlus northropi* (Wikimedia)

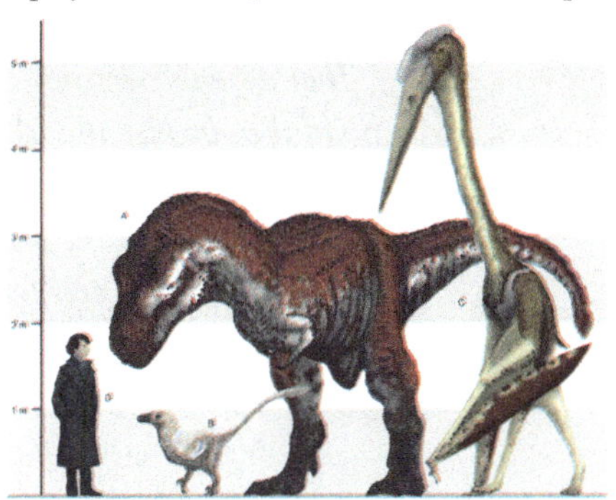

Quetzalcoaltus northropi vs. *Tyrannosaurus rex* (Wikimedia)
Witton, M. P., & Naish, D. (2015) Azhdarchid pterosaurs: Water-trawling pelican mimics or "terrestrial stalkers"? *Acta Palaeontologica Polonica*, 60(3), 651-660.

The Mesoamerican holocaust occurred in the decades overlapping those when Shakespeare wrote most of his legendary plays. Of course, no one in the Bard's world was the least bit aware of the disastrous consequences in the New World that were ignited by Columbus's arrival, which occurred only one hundred years before Shakespeare began to write. What Shakespeare and his contemporaries *did* comprehend, however, was the cataclysm ignited by the 1603 death of Queen Elizabeth I—Shakespeare's patron, his regent, his creative provocatrice, and certainly one of the pivotal monarchs in British history. In one of Shakespeare's two final plays, co-written with John Fletcher after Elizabeth's death, the Bard invokes the myth of the phoenix to describe Elizabeth's death and legacy. (Ironically, during the third performance of this play, the Globe theater was burned to the ground by the mis-fire of a prop cannon. However, the Globe soon rose from its ashes and roared back to life.)

Shakespeare's phoenix in this soliloquy is female, but his account of a "bird of wonder" who perishes in the flame and rises to redeem a nation could easily describe the spirit of Quetzalcoatl in Mesoamerica:

...But as when
The bird of wonder dies, the maiden phoenix,
Her ashes new create another heir,
As great in admiration as herself;
So shall she leave her blessedness to one,
When heaven shall call her from this cloud of darkness,

Who from the sacred ashes of her honor
Shall star-like rise, as great in fame as she was,
And so stand fix'd: peace, plenty, love, truth, terror,
That were the servants to this chosen infant,
Shall then be his, and like a vine grow to him:
Wherever the bright sun of heaven shall shine,
His honor and the greatness of his name
Shall be, and make new nations: he shall flourish,
And, like a mountain cedar, reach his branches
To all the plains about him: our children's children
Shall see this, and bless heaven.

– William Shakespeare and John Fletcher,
The Life of King Henry VIII, **V.v**

The Mesoamerican people appeared to perish in the post-Columbian holocaust of pandemic and oppression. But true to the phoenix myth of Quetzalcoatl, the spirit and genes of those ancient people rose up and flourish today as the "children of the plumed serpent" in south-central Mexico. Evidently, that which cannot survive in matter may yet rise again, first in spirit and then in descendant substance, despite all laws and logic. The original Mesoamericans may have been incinerated by pestilence and persecution, but their living legacy has risen from those ashes.

Meaningful Consequences from the 1918 Influenza Pandemic

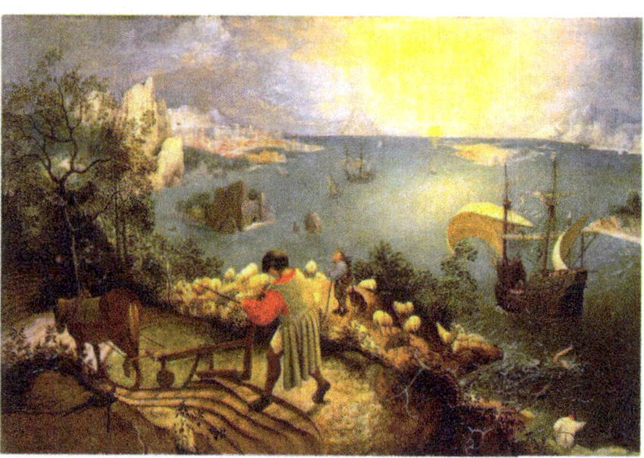

Landscape with the Fall of Icarus (1560) Pieter Brueghel the Elder
Royal Museums of Fine Arts of Belgium (Wikipedia)

About suffering they were never wrong,
The Old Masters: how well they understood
Its human position: how it takes place
While someone else is eating or opening a window
or just walking dully along...
In Breughel's Icarus, for instance: how everything turns away
Quite leisurely from the disaster; the ploughman may
Have heard the splash, the forsaken cry,
But for him it was not an important failure; the sun shone
As it had to on the white legs disappearing into the green
Water; and the expensive delicate ship, that must have seen
Something amazing, a boy falling out of the sky,
Had somewhere to get to and sailed calmly on.

– W. H. Auden (1939) "Musée des Beaux Arts"[138]

Simply because a disaster goes unnoticed in the moment that it happens, even if it goes unmentioned for decades thereafter, that doesn't lessen the disaster's tragedy. If anything, the fact that such anguish was less than ignored—was not even remarked—makes its calamity all the more profound, more poignant, and possibly more catastrophic. This, as we have learned, is the mystery and the tragedy of the 1918 influenza pandemic.

In reference to the painting and poem above...

A great artist does not often find artistic merit in commenting upon the work of another great artist, particularly when the commentary serves only to reiterate the essence of the original work. But the masterful W. H. Auden evidently found enormous importance in the subtle message of Brueghel's painting, and felt deep concern that the message itself would not be noticed, so much that he devoted a portion of his genius to articulating explicitly what Brueghel had depicted only implicitly. Perhaps Auden did not want Brueghel's experience (and others like it, including his own) to go as unremarked as the experience of Icarus.

In one sense, it is understandable why people would overlook the fall of Icarus. He wasn't anyone of particular note in Greco-Roman mythology—just a foolish boy by most accounts.[139] The more noteworthy character in Icarus's story, and in many others, was his father Daedalus—possibly the

138. Auden, Wystan Hugh. "Musée des Beaux Arts" in *Another Time*. New York: Random House, 1940. Copyright © 1939 by W.H. Auden. Reprinted by permission of Curtis Brown, Ltd. All rights reserved.

139. Ovid. *Metamorphoses*, Book 8. Translated by David Raeburn. New York: Penguin, 800/2004, pp. 307-312.

most gifted and famous craftsman of his age. Daedalus fabricated so many clever and beautiful things that all brilliant objects created in his time came to be known as *daidala*.

It is a curse, as well as a blessing, to be thus gifted. People who are similarly gifted know this all too well. Everyone loves the things that the artist creates, and we seem to love the artist for creating them. But then we come to realize that we are dependent on the artist when we yearn for something that doesn't yet exist. And we can also become frightened by the artist when we realize that such soaring creativity might work to our personal *dis*advantage.

This is exactly what happened to Daedalus in his relationship with King Minos, the powerful regent of Crete. Through a series of circumstances so unfortunate as to be nearly comic, the Queen of Crete fell in love with a sacred white bull that was given to Minos, with the intended purpose of serving as a sacrifice to the ocean god Poseidon. The Queen's bovine passion occurred because Minos offended Poseidon by deciding to keep the bull for himself. So Poseidon punished Minos by afflicting his Queen with a sexual obsession for the bull. Finding herself mad with passion, the Queen convinced (or maybe forced) Daedalus to create a way for her to mate with the bull. (Yes, these are the things that happen in the religious stories of ancient Greece. Which is why it's worth doing your mythology homework in high school.)

As luck (not the good kind) would have it, the mating of Queen and bull produced a terrible offspring...a child who was born with the body of a human and the head of a bull. The Queen called him Minotaur, explicitly naming after her husband this offspring of her escapade with the bull. (Complicated marital relations are *not* a modern invention.)

The Minotaur was problematic enough as a child, but once he matured to adulthood, he was dangerous beyond all managing. And yet, because he was the offspring of the Queen and a sacred animal, he could not be killed without Olympian consequences. So Minos hired Daedalus to build a "home" for the Minotaur—a dwelling in which the monster could roam around but never leave. And that is what Daedalus did. He built what has sometimes been called a maze, but was actually a *labyrinth*...a series of circular passages with no dead ends, but with such complexity that Daedalus himself nearly got lost within it. And thus the Minotaur was safely contained, endlessly wandering the concentric circles of the labyrinth.

Minos was deeply grateful to Daedalus...at first. But in the timeless tradition of faithful servants and fickle monarchs, Daelalus again found himself in the King's distrust, so he was imprisoned in a tall tower, along with his son Icarus. And this is where our story begins.

The tactic of locking up a clever person with nothing more on his hands than endless time and a determination to escape has led to all manner of brilliant strategies for liberation, ranging from Victor Hugo's *Count of Monte Cristo* to Stephen King's *The Shawshank Redemption*. In the story of Daedalus and his son, the escape strategy entailed the invention of wings. Specifically, these were two pairs of giant wings that Daedalus fabricated with *real* feathers...and quite cleverly so. They started with the smallest feathers near the shoulders and sloped to the largest feathers near the hands, just as a bird's are arranged. Daedalus made his wings with wax to bind the feathers to the frames, and straps to bind the frames to shoulders and hands.

He first tried out his own pair of wings, maneuvering them as a bird would into the winds that blew constantly at the top of the tower. Slowly, as he beat the great wings, Daedalus lifted into the air. The wings worked! He then tied the second pair of wings onto Icarus, and showed him how to move them to achieve the same lift. When the boy became excited with the feeling of becoming airborne, Daedalus spoke a severe warning: "My son! Do not fly too low, or the sea will wet the feathers and they will no longer lift you. And most importantly, *do not fly too high*, or the sun will melt the wax that binds the feathers together, and you will fall to your death!" And with that, Daedalus and his young Icarus spread their wings, lifted into the wind, and sailed toward freedom, away from their oppression and despair.

Even after we have spent decades being carried by metal airplane wings over oceans and continents, we can still imagine how thrilling that first flight must have been. And for the ancient Greeks, who could only *dream* of flying, the notion of taking off with Daedalus and his vibrant son must have seemed a kind of ecstasy. Indeed, the story does imply that this moment was ecstatic, both for the story's listeners and for its characters. It was astonishing enough for old Daedalus, with his time-worn decades of living. But for young Icarus, the rapture of flight was bedazzling. Higher and higher he flew, away from the imprisoning tower, away from the dousing waves, and away from his father's cries of increasing urgency and warning. Earth belonged to Icarus for those glorious minutes—a toy world to play with, a world all his own.

When did Icarus realize what was happening? Or did he ever realize the truth, blinded as he was by the sun's radiance? At what moment does one perceive that an ascent to one's victorious aspirations has become a descent to one's catastrophic demise? Perhaps one only awakens to the truth in the final moments. Or perhaps there are cases when one never awakens at all. It is all a glorious arc of power and freedom, soaring in triumph over land and sea, beyond humanity and mortality. Soaring faster and faster, higher and higher, until the larger forces of nature—the same forces that made the flight possible—demand that Nature's laws be heeded *in total.*

The wax began to melt under the watchful sun, and the feathers began to loosen from the wings. And whether or not he realized his imminent fate, once the remaining feathers touched the sea, Icarus was doomed. Daedalus, too, was doomed...to anguish. He could only watch the lightning descent of his beloved son, flashing past in a white blaze of flailing wings and widening eyes.

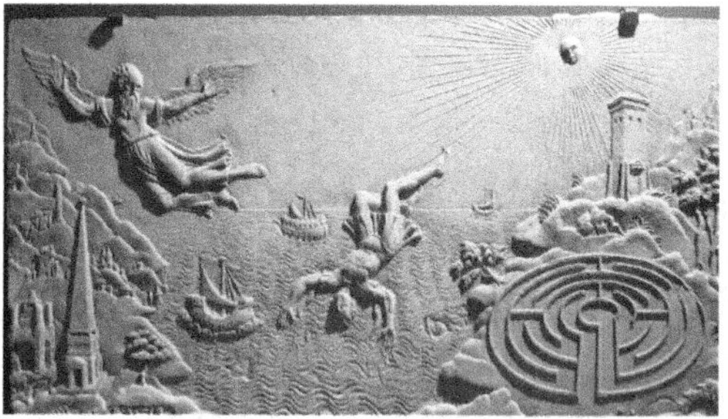

The Fall of Icarus (17th c. CE) Artist unknown (Musée Antoine Vivenel) (Wikimedia)

The story of Daedalus continued long after he witnessed the death of his son. His own flight ended successfully and he went on to design and create many more wondrous objects, becoming the Da Vinci of his time. But none of Daedalus's creations were worth as much to him as his precious son, whose body he buried on a nearby island. Daedalus named the island after Icarus, and it bears his name to this day...Icaria. Greek mythology tells us that Athena eventually took pity on Daedalus and granted him real wings, enabling him to truly fly. But we can imagine that no aeronautic gift could compensate for the loss that Daedalus had incurred by sharing his talent with his precious boy.

It would be nearly two thousand years after Ovid recounted the mythic flight of Icarus before Orville and Wilbur Wright would emulate his audacity at Kitty Hawk—with much more prudence and success, but with no less courage. And little more than ten years after that, the Allied and Central powers of Europe embarked on "the war to end all wars"—World War I. Three years later, in April 1917, the United States joined that gruesome enterprise. And in the following year of 1918, all the combatants in that war found themselves doing battle with a new enemy of a force that was superior to all of theirs combined—*influenza H1N1.* As we now know, the flu proved to be the ultimate victor in that war, claiming more than 50 million lives, as compared to the 10 million (or fewer) soldiers who died by combat.

But before *influenza H1N1* crashed their bloody party, the human participants in this global fiasco were filled with the same bold audacity that propelled Daedalus and Icarus when they leapt into the wind from their tower. The early 20th century was a period as complex as any in history, but one of its distinguishing traits was the blazing grandiosity of the Western peoples who were enjoying the benefits of the Industrial Revolution. Steam engines, telegraphs, and all manner of marvelous machines, including planes, trains, and automobiles. But especially those *aeroplanes*! World War I gave humans their first opportunity to deploy flight in the service of war. Biplanes couldn't achieve the lethality that bombers would later inflict, but the soaring aerobatics of the dogfighters evoke unmistakably the airborne euphoria of Icarus.

And it wasn't only the Allies. It was combatants on all sides of the war. Western civilization was blindly infatuated with its own invincibility, and its infatuation was hugely augmented by the juggernaut of its mechanized servants. We could now command powerful machines to help us kill our enemies (as well as drafting powerful animals for that same task, including the eight million horses, mules, and donkeys who died in our service during this "final" war).

It is possible that no war had ever been undertaken with such a meteoric confidence, nor shackled to such a massive deadweight of vulnerability. Our confidence was placed in lofty ideas, bold ambitions, and novel technologies, while our vulnerability huddled quietly in the merciless laws of Nature. It all resembled the lofty ideas, bold ambitions, and brilliant technology of a talented Greek father who crafted a way to defy both gravity and his King, and the fate of his son who joined his audacious campaign and who perished in the quirky and merciless grip of Nature.

Ten million soldiers fell from the heights of their leaders' soaring ambitions during World War I. But far beyond that, between 50 and 100 million people around the world crashed out of life as a result of the rampant flu pandemic—a pandemic whose danger was not only dismissed by the ambitious leaders, but was actually fanned into a deadly firestorm by their politics and the migrations of their war. The millions of flu victims were mostly uncounted when they died, and they remain uncountable to this day because of the fifty-year lag before they were noticed by *anyone*...except those who mourned them and the few artists who memorialized them at the time.

Well after all, who noticed Icarus as he fell? Only Daedalus—the father who loved him. Daedalus probably mourned his loss alone, feeling that he bore the guilt for Icarus's death. Mind you, many scholars during the past two millennia have assigned that guilt to Icarus, even though it is not clear that Ovid did so in his original poem. The story of Icarus is often held up as an example of *hubris*—a sin in ancient Greece of lethally exaggerated pride, in which a human would dare to defy or emulate the gods. Trying to outrun a divine prophecy (like Oedipus did), or trying to imitate divine powers (like flying with man-made wings) would certainly count for the ancient Greeks as sins of *hubris*. And such sins almost always led to very bad ends. But one might observe, and rightly so, that the actual *hubris* belonged to Daedalus, when he designed and donned the wings. Icarus only overshot the mark (or the altitude) in his fateful ascent, but he was otherwise being an obedient son, which usually earned the praise of the gods.

Now let's return to the story of World War I—that ghastly orgy of arrogance and aggression, in which all the combatants strutted their newfound status as global powers and flexed their recently-industrialized muscles in the exercise of war. Countless captains of invention and industry launched young people into their god-like plans, arming them with the treacherous miracles of poison gas, war engines, and flying machines. They crammed them into barracks, boats, bunkers, and stinking trenches, until it was only a matter of time before Nature added her own weaponry to the dreadful concoction—the weapon of contagion—which had appeared in many wars before this one, but never quite as effectively.

Well, this was the first war following the Industrial Revolution, was it not? Evidently, Nature became industrious, too, arriving in the war armed with H1N1 and claiming more victims than any other combatant. Her viral weapon was especially good at bringing down people who were young and strong, those who were just launching themselves into life. They fell from the skies, from their horses, from their feet, and from their lives. They fell directly into their graves, and only the people who had loved those flu victims seem to have mourned or remembered them.

As Icarus disappeared beneath the ocean waves and was buried on a tiny island in the Aegean Sea, so those millions of influenza victims disappeared beneath the waves of war news, to be buried later, and namelessly, beneath the mountains of peace negotiations, post-war rebuilding, the roaring 20s, the Great Depression, World War II, and a future obsessed with its own priorities. Only when another outbreak of Nature's viral fire—HIV/AIDS—began to claim the lives of strong young people in the 1980s, did the world return to examine the story of all those Icaruses who had been felled by flu during 1918-19.

The first and most obvious of the meaningful consequences from the 1918 influenza pandemic is the undisputed fact that it brought about the end of World War I, long before that bloody mess would have otherwise concluded. But beyond that, there is this ominous consequence...

In general, historians agree that the severe post-WWI hardships in Germany, which undoubtedly contributed to the rise of the Nazis, were fallout from the Treaty of Versailles, a retaliatory document that contained the infamous "war guilt clause," which falsely assigned to Germany *all* responsibility for the war and its damages.

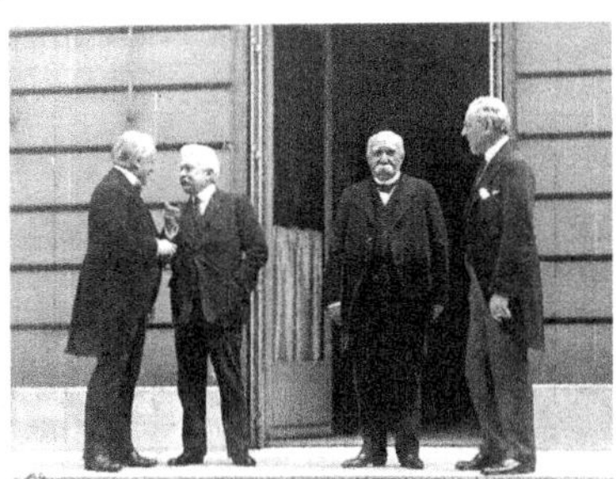

Lloyd George, Orlando, Clemenceau, and Wilson at Versailles (May 27, 1919) (Wikimedia)

The punitive measures contained in that Treaty were supposed to have been tempered by the U.S. President Woodrow Wilson. However, the Treaty became a vengeful whipping rod in the hands of the European allies—David Lloyd George for the United Kingdom, Vittorio Orlando for Italy, and Georges Clemenceau for France—because Wilson was disastrously incapacitated by the flu upon his arrival at the Paris summit.[140] Without Wilson's moderating influence, the resulting Treaty punished Germany brutally for a war that was *not* primarily of its making, and the Treaty's injustice made the "roaring 20s" a decade of bitter hardship for the German people. Quite plausibly, Hitler could not have roused the Germans to war again, only twenty years later, if the flu had not played this crucial role. We will never know for sure, but the hypothesis is widely held.

Beyond that hypothetical consequence of the H1N1 pandemic, it can be argued quite solidly that the post-WWI efforts made by medical researchers to solve the scientific mystery of the flu's lethality led to the identification of the virus in 1933, and much later, to the genomic sequencing of the 1918 version of H1N1. From that, it can be persuasively argued that had it not been for the 1918 flu and the research that proceeded from it, we might not be as far along in our knowledge of virology as we are today.

140. Barry, John M. *The Great Influenza: The Epic Story of the Deadliest Plague in History*. New York: Penguin, 2005.

In other words, were it not for the blinding lethality of H1N1, unremarked and unsung in its day but now recognized as the killer of millions (especially the young and the strong), who knows whether two determined scientists—Katalin Karikó and Drew Weissman—would have persisted so tenaciously in their determination to unlock the secrets of mRNA for viral vaccine delivery, which we recognize as the basis of today's most effective vaccines against novel coronavirus.[141]

Icarus was such a minor figure in Greco-Roman mythology that it is somewhat surprising that his story remains so well-known today. But from a Jungian perspective, the timeless durability of the Icarus story proves that his sad tale has always held great meaning for humankind. And why not? Given the millions of strong, bold, young people who have been felled throughout the centuries by their elders' audacious ambitions and the implacable forces of Nature, it is only reasonable that our hearts would resonate with a courageous young man who flew too near the sun, and with his horrified father who witnessed the tragic outcome of his overblown schemes.

Daedalus eventually resumed his creative workmanship, but we can imagine that Athena's gift of flight gave only slim solace to his grieving heart. And any ignorance, denial, or scapegoating of the tragedy was sure to increase the chances that its tragic consequences would be echoed into the future. Still, it is possible Daedalus's acts of creative penance may have led to more than even he could imagine in the way of healing the world.

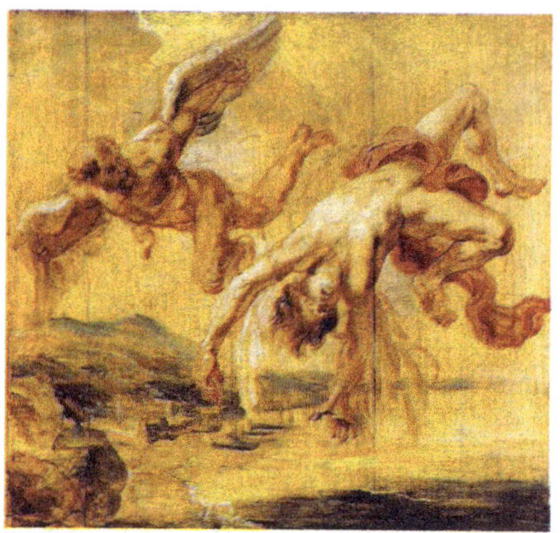

The Fall of Icarus (1635) Peter Paul Ruben (Wikimedia)

141. Short, Kirsty R., Katherine Kedzierska, and Carolien Van de Sandt. "Back to the Future: Lessons Learned from the 1918 Flu Pandemic" *Frontiers in Cellular and Infection Microbiology,* October 8, 2018. doi: 10.3389/fcimb.2018.00343

I see thy glory like a shooting star
Fall to the base earth from the firmament.
Thy sun sets weeping in the lowly west,
Witnessing storms to come, woe and unrest:
Thy friends are fled to wait upon thy foes,
And crossly to thy good all fortune goes.
– **William Shakespeare,** *Richard II,* **II.iv**

It would be so tempting at this point to embark on a spree of speculative pronouncements about the meaningful consequences that might proceed from the coronavirus pandemic. Unfortunately, a spree like that would require us to pretend that colorful conjectures are valid substitutes for the actual consequences and retrospective insights that can only emerge long after the pandemic we are evaluating.

Fortunately, a successful drama can declare some of its essential meaning long before its literal outcome. Indeed, a really well-written play declares its essence throughout its length, planting the seeds of its conclusion in the earliest lines of its major characters:

Now is the winter of our discontent
Made glorious summer by this son of York.
(*Richard III*)

Attend the lords of France and Burgundy, Gloucester.
Meantime we shall express our darker purpose.
(*King Lear*)

'Sblood, but you will not hear me:
If ever I did dream of such a matter, abhor me.
(**Iago in** *Othello*)

Therefore, as I have done throughout this book, I will treat the coronavirus pandemic as a play. Yes, it is a play whose final act has not yet been written, but enough of this drama has transpired so that we may be able to discern some of its essence in the lines we have already heard, in the characters we have already met, in the scenes we have already witnessed.

It is also true that stories and characters tend to repeat themselves over the course of centuries. Even Shakespeare based his iconic works on the stories he found in the annals of history, as well as the timeless characters he observed in the world around him. So I will look for the common themes between the coronavirus pandemic and the historical pandemics, seeking some sense of consequence for the current pandemic from among the meaningful consequences to pandemics that have gone before—pandemics that afflicted and transformed human beings who were very much like ourselves.

This final chapter will be an epilogue, an experiment of inference as well as deduction. Let's see if Polyhymnia, the Greek muse who presided over historical and imaginative storytelling, can bring forth a glimmer of meaning from our shadowy future in the tale of the coronavirus pandemic—a story whose ending has yet to be revealed.

EPILOGUE

Possible Consequences of Meaning from the Coronavirus Pandemic

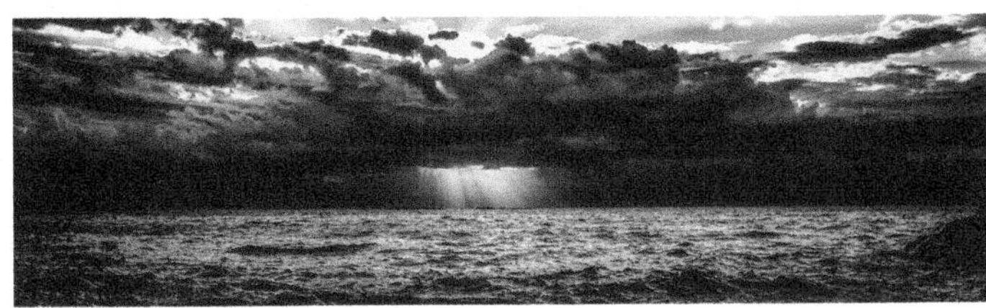

(Shutterstock)

When you come out of the storm,
you won't be the same person who walked in.
That's what the storm is all about.
– Haruki Murakami[142]

A story only matters, I suspect, to the extent
that the people in the story change.
– Neil Gaiman[143]

A century (or four) from now, some clever historian will be able to draw all sorts of insightful conclusions about the meaningful consequences that have emerged from the coronavirus pandemic. But most of us would like to have a whiff of those conclusions a little sooner than a century (or four) from now. Probably, we would like to get that whiff within our own lifetimes, or better yet, within the next half hour. And most of us would like to have more than a "whiff" of the meaningful consequences that are likely to emerge from this viral bonfire. Specifically, we would like a clear sense about how the Covid pandemic is changing our world, changing our lives, and changing each of us in ways that we hope will be positive, important, and enduring.

The difficulty in obtaining this vision of the future might make us yearn for that DeLorean with the flux-capacitor. But the truth is that we will probably derive more pandemic insight from scrutinizing the past than from

142. Murakami, Haruki. *Kafka on the Shore.* New York: Knopf Doubleday, 2006.
143. Gaiman, Neil. *The Ocean at the End of the Lane.* New York: William Morrow, 2019.

speculating about the future. This coronavirus may be novel, but the human beings it is killing, infecting, and otherwise distressing are not novel at all. Humankind's millennial history with pestilence has much to say about how the coronavirus pandemic is likely to transform us and our world.

Throughout this book, we have examined the dramas of four major pandemics in human history, and each of them has shown us a different narrative with a unique cast of characters. But we have also found several common elements among those four pandemics—some elements that we may have expected and others that took us by surprise. Considered together, these common elements create a pretty cohesive pattern of the effects that pandemics have had on our species.

Let's integrate those common elements from past pandemics and see if we can create a platform on which we can stand, so that we might compose a few meaningful consequences that the coronavirus pandemic is likely to have for our frail but ferocious species.

Common Consequences from the Historical Pandemics

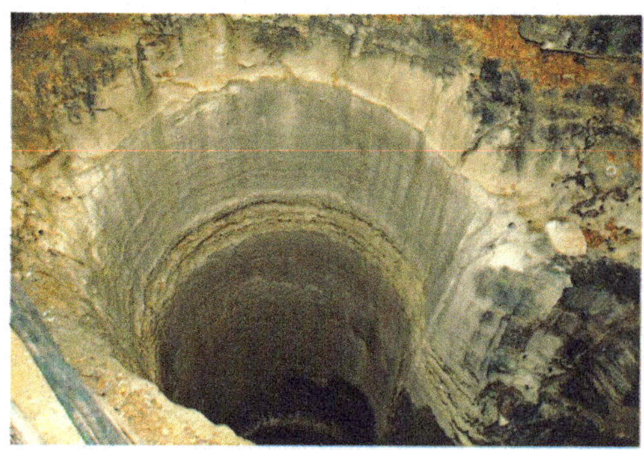

(Wikimedia)

It is by going down into the abyss
that we recover the treasures of life.
– Joseph Campbell[144]

If you gaze long enough into an abyss,
the abyss will gaze back into you.
– Friedrich Nietzsche[145]

144. Campbell, Joseph. *A Joseph Campbell Companion.* New York: Harper Perennial, 24.

145. Friedrich Nietzsche. "Chapter IV: Apophthegms and Interludes, §146" in *Beyond Good and Evil: Prelude to a Philosophy of the Future.* https://www.gutenberg.org/files/4363/4363-h/4363-h.htm#link2HCH0004

Beneath the unique experiences that our species has endured through the historical pandemics, there are six common themes that we can discern in their dramas:

1. The invading diseases of our pandemics have always taken us by surprise, usually raising our alarms only after they have gravely infected our populations.
2. The micro-defenders of our immune systems have responded with fierce consistency to Nature's pestilential protagonists. But when those micro-defenders have not been able to drive off these disease invaders (as they have not in the case of global pandemics), it is our innate immune systems themselves that have been the primary causes of our suffering and death.
3. The battles between humanity and its diseases have primarily been fought on this microscopic level, even as our macroscopic brains have consistently dismissed and disrespected the microscopic world...at the cost of our terrible suffering.
4. Our behavioral responses to our micro-invaders have also been fiercely consistent across the millennia. Our urges toward denial, regression, projection, and magical thinking have competed with our capacities for logic, preparation, wit, and sublimation. Some of us have mustered the sterling traits of stoicism, pragmatism, and compassion in the presence of a pandemic, while others of us have always fallen into self-absorption, reactivity, and scapegoating.
5. The effect of pandemic disease on the collective human psyche has always been to precipitate our descent into a darker realm of consciousness. Individuals and societies who have been afflicted by pestilence have entered a twilight region of retreat and uncertainty, a netherworld of grief for everything that has been lost, a shadowy cave of profound disorientation, desperate survival, and looming despair. And yet, it seems that this dark place has always offered its survivors the seeds of truth, with a potential of redemption for future generations.
6. Eventually (and this outcome may take years or even centuries), the survivors of each pandemic drama have returned from their descent. Consciously or not, they have been deeply changed by their cloistered time of pandemic withdrawal, while the world itself has been changed by the cataclysm of pestilence. Much has been lost, but something has always been gained, especially by

> those who have planted and nurtured those seeds of truth and redemption. This is where the next act of our human drama has always begun, once the pandemic has subsided.

Now let's take a quick look at the ways these six elements seem to be playing out in the drama of the coronavirus pandemic, and perhaps we will discern some patterns that suggest how this pandemic will change us and our world, hopefully in meaningful ways.

#1—Protagonist Diseases Always Take Us By Surprise[146]

Surprises are foolish things.
The pleasure is not enhanced, and the
inconvenience is often considerable.
– Jane Austen

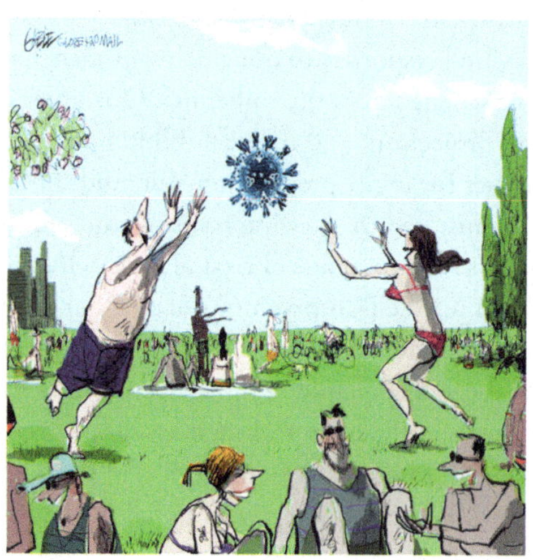

© 2020 Brian Gable, *The Canadian Globe and Mail*

It wasn't only Donald Trump who was blind-sided by the speed and virulence of the novel coronavirus. In retrospect, it is clear that the Chinese authorities grossly underestimated the grave peril that this virus posed when it was first

146. © 2020 Brian Gable, *The Canadian Globe and Mail.* Originally published May 14, 2020. Reprinted by permission of The Canadian Press Enterprises, Inc.

detected inside their borders.[147] And their disastrous error in judgment was quickly repeated by the authorities in nearly every country of the world. Most leaders responded so slowly and ineffectually, and in some cases so dishonestly, that the virus had planted its microscopic flag around the globe before anyone sounded an alarm that was proportionate to its danger.

Even when that alarm was sounded, it took a remarkably long time for humanity to give credence to the threat. This delay is especially impressive when we consider that those of us in first-world countries are accustomed to responding at the speed of electrons. We can pivot on the pinpoint of a Tweet when we read about possible contaminants in our cat food. But we couldn't seem to muster an adrenal nudge, let alone a pinpoint pivot, in response to news about the imminent arrival of a human virus with deadly tactics of colonization.

This "taken by surprise" factor is probably related to one common characteristic of pandemic disease, which is the fact that global pandemics don't actually happen all that often. Yes, the Black Death lasted four hundred years, but it had erupted in Europe nearly eight hundred years after the Plague of Justinian. And after the Black Death had burned through Europe for the final time, it would be two hundred more years before the H1N1 influenza virus pandemic began its deadly campaign of world conquest. So we might be somewhat forgiven for our sluggish response to an invader whose assaults occur so infrequently.

And of course, there's that invisibility factor. Even though humanity can now use electron microscopes to see the pathogens that mow us down by the millions, those bugs are still invisible to the naked eye. This makes it hard for us to take them as seriously as an enemy the size of Godzilla. Several millennia and many pandemics after our earliest encounters with these micro-invaders, we still act as if size matters...and as if tiny size *doesn't* matter. Tell that to SARS-CoV-2. The joke's on us, my macro-centric friends.

Finally, we children of the 20th and 21st centuries have a particular disadvantage when it comes to giving to pandemic diseases the terrified respect that they deserve. No first-world person alive today remembers the time when vaccination was a rare and precious privilege, the time when we were afflicted and killed by many dreadful diseases we can now prevent by vaccination. The annual summer outbreaks of polio are relics of medical history, as are mass eruptions of measles, mumps, whooping cough, diphtheria, and rubella. Even chicken pox is receding as a common affliction (and frequent

147. Editorial Board of *The Washington Post*. "As the pandemic exploded, a researcher saw the danger. China's leaders kept silent." *Washington Post*, April 22, 2022. https://www.washingtonpost.com/opinions/interactive/2022/china-researcher-covid-19-coverup/

killer) of humanity. And, of course, the "speckled monster" of smallpox is extinct. This "out of sight, out of mind" bias has deadly implications. Nestled in our manufactured haven of vaccine protection, we have come to believe that we can rebuff nearly all contagious diseases as long as we exercise regularly, take our vitamins, and eat lots of kale.

This belief has led some of us to conclude that vaccination is now irrelevant, and even detrimental, as compared to the diseases that it holds at bay. That attitude is essentially a form of narcissism that wraps its believers in a delusion of dominance over Nature's micro-citizens. The delusion may be comforting, but it is very dangerous because when we receive word of a new disease, it is hard for our deluded selves to believe that the tiny newcomer could easily become a mass murderer. Of course, there have been some very smart people who have been warning us that the Horseman of Pestilence could ride again, quite suddenly and without any notice. But it is always so hard to take pestilence seriously...not until it is actively demolishing the soft flesh of our good fortune and good health.

For all these reasons, we heedless humans are always taken by surprise when Pestilence crashes our comfortable parties, tramples our familiar routines, shatters our cherished expectations, and abducts us into a realm that is ominous, unpredictable, and riven with change. When pandemic disease strikes, we are like Persephone and Dante—abducted without warning into a netherworld of uncertainty. And no matter what encouraging tune we whistle to ourselves in that grave place, we have a gnawing dread that life will never be the same again. Our dread is quite correct. Certain elements of living may stay constant after the conflagration of pestilence has subsided. But life as we knew it will be changed forever. Like Icarus, we have been felled from our lofty plans, and plunged into depths that could end all of our dreams. We have a deep sense that this conflagration of contagion might incinerate us, like Quetzalcoatl and his phoenix kin. And in the wildfire of pandemic disease, we could be right.

Every pandemic assault, and every subsequent descent into the black realm of loss, comes upon us by surprise. Every pandemic. Every time. This coronavirus pandemic has been no exception. The dark netherworld is where we have been, where many of us still are, and where many of us will remain for a much longer time than we are willing to believe. In the fall of 2021, we watched the "delta" variant of the virus drive a surge of infection and death through a world that was minimally vaccinated, even as many privileged people were adamantly refusing vaccination. In 2022, we have watched the "omicron" variant sweep the world with a new wave of illness. At this point, we can only hope that future pandemic historians will say that this pandemic taught us to be less obtuse, less distracted, less willfully disdainful of the danger posed by pathogenic invaders. But that hope is not being supported by current human behavior.

It will be way beyond tragic if we are to succumb to yet another viral ambush as a result of our own stubborn narcissism. To quote Louis Pasteur once again, "Fortune favors the prepared." And surprise favors only the attacker. We have no excuse for being surprised at this point. And at our current densities of global population, speeds of global transportation, and inequities of global resources, we can no longer afford this habit of pathogenic disregard. Awakening to the catastrophic danger of pestilence, and responding to it in a proactive way, could be a deeply meaningful consequence of this pandemic, a transformative bit of progress for the human race. On the other hand, our stubborn refusal to accept and play by Nature's rules for pandemic disease could place our burgeoning populations in extreme peril. Can we change our human ways?[148]

#2—The micro-antagonists of our immune systems have always defended us in the same ways against pandemic pathogens. Their methods are remarkably efficient and elegant, but when our innate immune systems fail to drive off the invaders (as they always have failed in global pandemics), our immune systems themselves become the primary causes of our suffering and death.

First, the simplest and most important fact. Without our innate immune systems—the micro-defenders who are our fastest and most efficient weapons against the determined invaders of pandemic disease—we would be dead almost as soon as we drew breath. Even the advanced weaponry of vaccination is merely a means of giving our adaptive immune system a turbo-boost to enhance its latent talent for killing a specific disease before it kills us. As impressive as our massive brains might be, our immune systems have the millennial advantage of evolutionary refinement, as well as the capacity to engage those determined micro-protagonists on their own microscopic terms. The best our forebrains can do is to comprehend those micro-terms

148. The Editorial Board of the *Washington Post*. "The Coming Storm: America is not ready for a future pandemic." *Washington Post*, August 27, 2022. https://www.washingtonpost.com/outlook/2022/08/25/long-covid-brain-science-fog-recovery/

and devise macro-methods for supporting them—methods like social distancing, hygiene protocols, and of course, vaccination.

Without the life-saving element of vaccination, the techniques of masking, maximal hygiene, social distancing, and quarantine are our only means of fending off pandemic invaders. These techniques have historically ranged from being moderately effective to tragically useless, depending on the disease and the circumstances. And when these macro-measures of prevention fail, leaving our innate immune systems to fight as best they can in the absence of vaccination, it is their own valiant actions that usually lead to our deaths.

This is why the deployment of anticipation and preparation, coupled with the scientific method, have been revolutionary in reducing the death counts from pandemic disease. Preventative measures, especially vaccine development, are crucial in the control of pestilence, because pandemic diseases are exactly the ones that confound our innate immune systems, leading them to burn down the homes of our bodies while they vainly try to burn up the home invaders of disease.

#3—Despite their primacy and constancy, we have always disrespected the laws of the natural world, especially the laws of the microscopic worlds within us and around us.

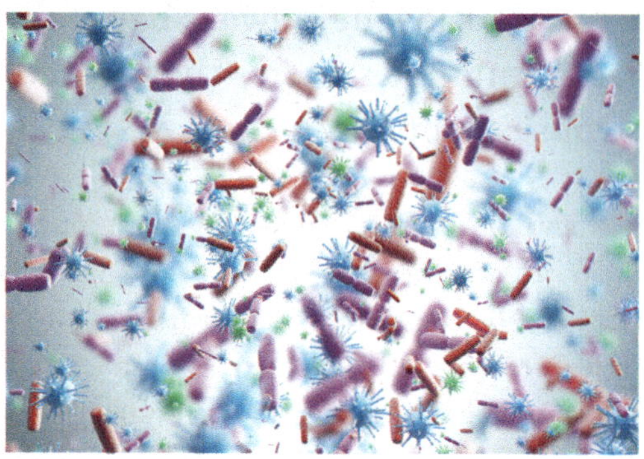

A depiction of our microscopic world (Shutterstock)

And this our life, exempt from public haunt,
Finds tongues in trees, books in the running brooks,
Sermons in stones, and good in everything.
– William Shakespeare, ***As You Like It***, II.i

Nature always bats last.
– Robert K. Watson[149]

The advantage of our massive brains is that they enable us to devise the tactics of prevention. The challenge is that in order for our brains to devise these tactics, they have to set aside the bias of our large human dimensions and surrender to the laws of the microscopic realm in which our pestilential invaders and our immunological defenders must do battle. This micro-view is a difficult mindset for us to maintain when we are juggling school lunches, work deadlines, and dental appointments. We are, after all, macroscopic creatures in body and mind, and it cramps our self-image (not to mention our self-esteem) to reorganize our lives by microscopic rules.

But here's the bottom line... *All of Nature operates according to microscopic rules.* Every virus and every volcano is microscopically driven, and every light bulb, automobile, plastic bottle, and human being is a contributing member on the microscopic level. Sadly, we only notice the microscopic effects of an object when they accumulate to macroscopic proportions, just as we only notice the microscopic invasions of pandemic pathogens when they accumulate to macroscopic symptoms in our bodies. We don't notice microscopic things unless we have to...or occasionally, in a moment of blessed awakening, when we *choose* to.

But mostly, we ignore what we cannot easily see, and we *really* ignore what we don't want to see. For some reason, the microscopic laws of Nature have mostly fallen into our don't-want-to-see category. Monumental tomes have been written to explain this self-defeating quirk in humanity's denial of Nature. But I prefer to cut through such bulky explanations with Occam's razor. That is, when I hear hoofbeats, I think horses, not zebras. The simplest explanation for our persistent, even stubborn, refusal to acknowledge and embrace Nature's laws is that Nature confuses, overwhelms, and intimidates us.

It's not that we humans are being intentionally perverse when we insist that we can dominate Nature. It's just that we're so very *tiny* in comparison to the great all-ness of everything else. And that reality is too painful for most of us to acknowledge, let alone embrace. I mean, just try to think about the Universe, for starters, which is too big to even be considered, let alone comprehended. And then consider things like earthquakes and

149. Robert Watson is a famous environmental architect quoted by Thomas Friedman in "We're gonna be sorry." *The New York Times*, July 24, 2010. https://www.nytimes.com/2010/07/25/opinion/25friedman.html

forest fires and gravity and rattlesnakes, which are daunting enough when taken by ones and twos, but simply mind-blowing when taken altogether as Nature's bounty. So by the time we get down to the microscopic things like bacteria and viruses and fractiles of synchronistic effect, we are left with nothing but the wispy vapors of our fleeting human existence. Out, brief candle!

Or else...

We can pretend that the whole of Nature's show is ours to explore, enjoy, and exploit. Or at the very least, we can pretend that it's ours to manage and manipulate to our own purposes. And this is what we mostly do, what we have mostly done for millennia. This is the same human audacity that has led humankind, alone among all species, to fight back against pandemic disease. It's a kind of bravado that has to be admired...but only up to a point. Because it's an illusion, of course. We don't control Nature and Nature's rules. We only use those rules to serve our chosen ends. And while we're using those rules, we *pretend* that we're the ones in control, for the purposes of speed and self-esteem. Our pretense functions well enough...as long as we don't push Nature's rules past their limits. But if we don't acknowledge that those rules come from forces larger than our human egos, we probably won't acknowledge their limits. And the harsh truth about pushing Nature's rules beyond their limits is that those rules always push *back*.

True, they don't always push back at the same speed. For example, let's say someone decides to push the law of gravity beyond a certain limit by jumping off a ten-story building with the hope of drifting to the ground like a feather. In that case, gravity is going to push back immediately, and hard. But if someone decides that they're going to push the limits of the viral contagion rules by declaring that "I don't believe in the novel coronavirus!"... well, it is possible that the virus might not push back right away. The viral rule-pusher might possibly be fine for a while, but then find themselves being hooked to a ventilator and begging in vain for a vaccine. And that's the first time they will realize that although they didn't believe in the novel coronavirus, the novel coronavirus always believed in *them*.

Waking up to the hard truth about Nature's laws and realities requires a profound remodeling of one's world view. It doesn't matter whether or not we "believe in" Nature and the sciences that study Nature. The bottom line is that Nature believes in *us*...every single one of us, every single second. Nature's rules apply without relenting, without exception, and without hard feelings. Gravity pulls down, viruses replicate, and immune systems overreact. Those are just the rules of physics, biology, and chemistry. Their primacy is a simple fact. But the facts of Nature's primacy seem always to be daunting to our brief and tender psyches. Sadly, if we don't embrace Nature's authority, our brief and tender lives become much briefer. And much less tender. Embracing Nature's primacy may be hard, but it's necessary for a successful human existence.

And this is where the netherworld becomes relevant...

In all four of the mythic stories we have linked to the historical pandemics—Persephone, Dante, Quetzalcoatl, and Icarus—the hero's descent into darkness led to a dramatic change in perspective and a fundamental shift in consciousness. Although our human descents during global pandemics have always been metaphorical and mostly unconscious, they seem to have produced similar kinds of shifts and changes in consciousness. Yes, the changes were usually subtle, incremental, and very slow. But they were also profound and lasting.

Our descent in the coronavirus pandemic has mostly been metaphorical and unconscious. It's been a descent from our upper-world macro-expectations about office work, classrooms, vacations, appointments, and next week's poker night. We've been forced to descend downward from the illusion that our most dangerous opponents were a different political group, a restrictive credit limit, an ignorant supervisor, or a regressive social norm. Suddenly, our greatest enemy has become something so small that a billion of them could share the pinpoint upon which we just refused to pivot. Nearly all of us have found this descent to be frightening, destabilizing, and, finally, exhausting. Eventually, some of us have discovered hidden resources of quietude and calm after we were forcibly sequestered in our Covid-prevention shelters. But others of us have remained distraught and depressed, stalking the perimeters of our sheltered spaces like terrified animals who have fallen into the trap of a narrow abyss. The micro-perspective is not equally illuminating to us all.

Or perhaps it would be more accurate to say that the micro-perspective is *differently* illuminating to different people. What some of us have found in that twilight netherworld is the deeper truth of our values and feelings. Given a choice between the illusion of security in a job we loathe and the acceptance of life's uncertainty in a different job we love, we are choosing the path of tangible risk and surprising reward. Workers throughout the Western world are changing vocations at record levels. Even the young people in work-driven China are selecting the life of *tangping* or "lying flat," in which they are rejecting consuming jobs, burdensome possessions, and obligatory relationships.[150] As Nature makes clear the fragility of life during this pandemic, many of us are adjusting our lives to honor the precious moments we have. We have evidence of this consequence from every historical pandemic, but it is important to note that it is becoming a consequence of the coronavirus pandemic, as well.

Others of us are deriving from our awakening to Nature's primal role a newfound awareness of ourselves as Nature's beings. This is similar to the profound transition that followed the Black Death, when Western society remembered that we humans are creatures of embodied Nature, even before we are spiritual acolytes. As Nature reminded us back then that we are embodied before we are anything else, so some of us have now awakened to the most primary natural elements of our bodies and the implications of those elements. Issues of ethnicity and gender/sexuality have long been simmering in the world, but the recent global explosion of racial outrage following the murder of George Floyd in America, and the congruent global explosion of gender/sexual consciousness, are similar to other movements of social progress that have followed global pandemics. When Nature loudly announces her primacy through a deadly pathogen, many of us answer her with equal assertiveness about the primacy of our *natures*. And that is only *natural*.

Pandemic disease forces us to remember that Nature is in charge, everywhere and all the time. Thanks to our massive brains and our genius for adapting, we humans have the privilege during healthier times of collaborating with Nature and soaring beyond our rudimentary origins. But when pathogenic protagonists arrive, we are once again reminded of our humble foundations—foundations that we have not left behind in some ancient pre-human ancestor, but rather, foundations that we carry in every living cell. Pandemics invite us to remember our microscopic origins, to recognize that those origins are with us still, and to realize that our origins can sustain and enhance our futures...but only if we respect their primacy and power.

Nature bats last, as she has always batted first, and we are all on Nature's team. If we play with her, we win. If we play against her, if we try to invent new rules, we will lose in the end...and badly. Respect for Nature, and for ourselves as Natural beings, could be another meaningful consequence of this pandemic. For the sake of our survival and well-being, I certainly hope it is.

150. Kuo, Lily. "Young Chinese take a stand against pressures of modern life—by lying down." *Washington Post*, June 5, 2021. https://www.washingtonpost.com/world/asia_pacific/china-lying-flat-stress/2021/06/04/cef36902-c42f-11eb-89a4-b7ae22aa193e_story.html

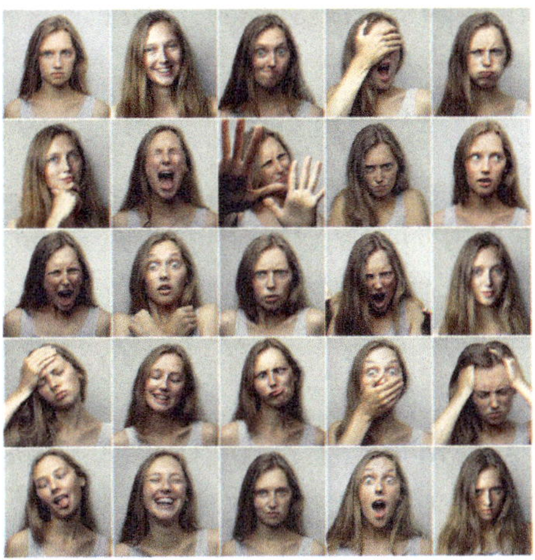

(Shutterstock)

#4—Our macro-defending responses to the stress of pandemic invaders have been consistent across the ages…both for the better and the worse.

CLOV: All life long the same questions, the same answers…

HAMM: Ah, the old questions, the old answers,
there's nothing like them!
– Samuel Beckett, *Endgame*[151]

Just as the human body is not a novel player in this story of the novel coronavirus, so our stress responses are not novel either. And just as our biological defenses are hard-wired into our organic beings, so our behavioral defenses emerge instinctively when we face a frightening invader. We have seen how dysfunctional, and even self-destructive, some of our responses can be in the fight against a micro-protagonist. Nonetheless, it is important to recognize the ways in which each of our macro-defenses can serve a particular purpose during a global pandemic:

Denial allows us keep functioning when we are confronted by pandemic disease, a terrifying threat that might freeze us solid with fear if we acknowledged its deadly reality.

151. Beckett, Samuel. *Endgame and Act Without Words*. New York: Grove Press, 1954/2009.

Regression permits us to behave as children do when they are protected from an imminent danger. We can delight in daily pleasures, pursue our cherished plans and projects without concern that they will be taken from us, and elaborate our dreams for the future without any worry that they will not come to life in due time. Hope is preserved, and with it, our proactive life force and creative capacities for problem-solving and surviving.

Magical Thinking enables us to engage the looming disease with bulletproof confidence. We arm ourselves with the astounding delusion that our fantasized powers of defense, and our equally fantastic delusions about the disease's frailty, will serve to keep us alive and healthy. It is pure fantasy, but it does keep us moving and breathing with confidence...until we die.

Displacement (Scapegoating) gives us a target to blame for the pestilence that has so unfairly and inconveniently ruptured our privileged and tranquil lives. If we cannot beat the virus to a pulp, we might get some compensatory satisfaction from inflicting similar damage—physical or emotional—on the people that we fantasize are to blame.

Projection permits us to transfer our intolerable feelings about the disease to someone else, preferably someone who seems to deserve them and who can't fight back. Finding other people who are terrified, mourning, or in despair (or inciting those feelings in other people) gives us a sense of relief and empowerment, even if it does nothing to fight the disease.

Repression empowers us to stifle our terror, grief, and/or despair in the midst of a pandemic, thereby allowing us to carry on in our normal lives and even perform acts of courage and compassion that place us in danger of contagion.

Identification gives us the ability to model our response to the disease based on the response of someone else...preferably someone who is responding more successfully than we might if we simply followed our own primitive instincts.

Rational analysis offers us the capacity to use our nimble minds and cool reason in the work of opposing the disease, thereby saving lives, health, and a measure of our own sanity in the midst of the panic and chaos.

Anticipation and preparation are the skills that prevent our being taken by surprise when the pathogen strikes, thereby improving our chances of quickly developing effective methods for combatting and defeating the invader.

Humor enables us to maintain a stable emotional footing and a larger perspective when we are confronted by a disease that would otherwise scare the peewonkers out of us. It also keeps our creativity engaged, which can improve our search for effective countermeasures.

Sublimation allows us to "see the cathedral in a pile of rocks," or more prosaically, to see the solution that resides within the problem. For example, every vaccine employs sublimation by using the pathogen's own genetic code as a training tool for our adaptive immune system.

Human beings have displayed some combination of these behaviors in response to our major stressors—pandemic and otherwise—ever since we began walking on our hind legs. For all we know, other primates (and perhaps some non-primate mammals) deploy some of these stress responses, too. The difference is that, unlike every other species, we humans have been displaying them in particular response to pandemic disease. And this wide range of responses has always had the same wide range of effects in combatting virulent disease, varying from "astoundingly successful" to "it probably would have been better to just lie down and die."

In the ages before microscopes and vaccination, it was only natural that we would resort to macro-defenses like scapegoating and endorsing magical thinking. Scapegoating minority groups is a timeless tactic for responding to all kinds of societal stressors. And archaic medicine was often synonymous with the fantastic (though ineffective) tactics of magical thinking. The astonishing thing about the coronavirus pandemic is that so many people have fiercely embraced these same stress responses of scapegoating (invoking "Democrat hoaxers" or "fascist allopaths") and magical remedies (like ingesting bleach or following a vegan diet), all of which are as useless in the fight against coronavirus as were the burning of Jewish towns and the wearing of bird-beaked masks in fighting the Black Death. This has been especially surprising in countries like America, where few people resist going to a medical doctor when they break their leg.

It would be easy to lay the responsibility for this unfortunate phenomenon at the feet of Donald Trump, with his endorsement of voodoo treatments and his dismissal of reputable medical advice. But the reality is part of a much larger phenomenon:

> "COVID-19 hit at an inauspicious geopolitical moment. An era of rising nationalism and populism made it frustratingly difficult to mount a collaborative response to a global pandemic. Jair Bolsonaro of Brazil, Xi Jinping of China, Narendra Modi of India, Vladimir Putin of Russia, Recep Tayyip Erdogan of Turkey, Boris Johnson of the United Kingdom, and Donald Trump of the United States—all these leaders evinced some

> combination of parochialism and political insecurity, which caused them to downplay the crisis, ignore the science, and reject international cooperation."[152]

This disparity of cultures, which we discussed regarding the "narrative" of the coronavirus pandemic, has deepened into a chasm of tragic conflict, not only in America but also in other Western countries. Vaccination and the preventative measures of masking and social distancing have become divisive political issues, rather than rational medical countermeasures. As this sociopolitical crevasse has become more extreme, so have the frequency of ineffective stress responses such as denial, regression, projection, and magical thinking. This situation exists in many countries, but nowhere is it as extreme as in the United States; as of April 2022, America still has the highest number of Covid cases and deaths in the world, despite having more resources per capita than any other country and far from having the largest national population.

It is impossible to say what the meaningful consequence of this dreadful statistic will be for America. But if anything can be said with fair confidence about the current consequences from the coronavirus pandemic, it is that they prove that the human response to any pathogenic protagonist must be immediate, honest, courageous, and fact-based if we are to prevail over a microscopic invader. To return to an earlier metaphor, fighting a pandemic is like fighting a forest fire. Denial, dawdling, dissembling, and disputing will result in nothing but cold ash...and a lot of it. Just ask the people in Narendra Modi's India, who were melting the pipes in their crematoria as they attempted to keep up with all the bodies that needed to be burned following the disastrous ignition of Covid in spring 2021—an ignition from the seething coals of contagion that were ignored, a conflagration that buried that country in the ashes of its dead.

On the other hand, the more we can emulate the rational, proactive conduct of the vaccine developers like Katalin Karikó, who began her mRNA researches *thirty years* before they were deployed for the Pfizer/BionTech and Moderna vaccines, the more likely we will be to prevail over the next pandemic protagonist. As we have been told (and most of us darkly suspect), the next protagonist could be a much more efficient serial killer than the merely appalling murderer that we are battling in SARS-CoV-2.

152. Brilliant, Larry, Lisa Danzig, Karen Oppenheimer, Agastya Mondal, and Rick Bright. "The Forever Virus: A Strategy for the Long Fight Against COVID-19." *Foreign Affairs* 100, no.4, July/August 2021. https://omnilogos.com/forever-virus-strategy-for-long-fight-against-covid19/

It is possible that this difference in human stress response patterns has never been as extreme during a global pandemic as it has been during this one. It remains to be seen whether the current contrast will result in a cataclysmic war of incompatible responses, or whether we will finally, as Rilke exhorts, manage to "take our practiced powers and spread them out until they span the chasm between two contradictions." If we accomplish the latter, if humankind manages to reconcile its primitive urges for denial, regression, and fantasy with its crucial need for fact-based analysis, preparation, and creative problem-solving, we may arrive at another of the most profound consequences in the history of human pandemics.

This lesson is waiting to be learned, and not only by those of us who are biochemists, but by all of us who care about avoiding another pandemic with a body count in the millions and a disability toll that is yet to be tallied.

#5—Pandemics force us to descend into a place of darkness, truth, and possible redemption.

(In my sleep I dreamed this poem)
Someone I loved once gave me
a box full of darkness.
It took me years to understand
that this, too, was a gift.

– Mary Oliver[153]

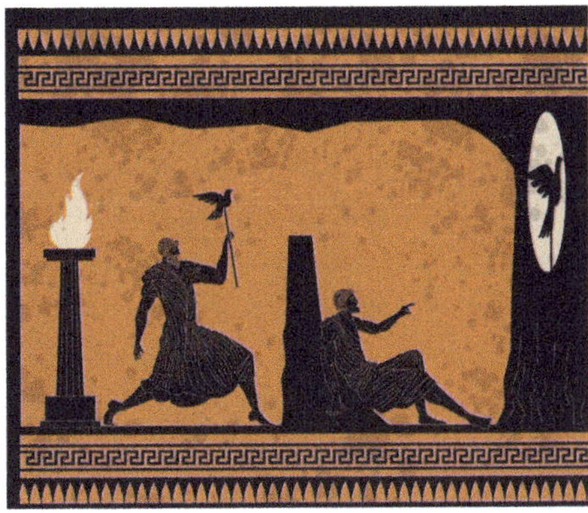

Plato's Cave, Matias Del Carmine (Shutterstock)

153. Oliver, Mary. "The Uses of Sorrow" in *Thirst.* New York: Beacon Press, 2007. Reprinted by the permission of The Charlotte Sheedy Literary Agency, LLC, as agent for the author. Copyright © 2006 by Mary Oliver with permission of Bill Reichblum.

In the four myths that I have invoked to capture the essences of the four historical pandemics—Persephone, Dante, Quetzalcoatl, and Icarus—the descents of the major characters were unforeseen, incomprehensible, and fairly traumatic. When people talk about their experience of the coronavirus pandemic, they seem to echo these mythic themes. Human beings of every gender, age, and ethnicity are describing the sense that they have been snatched out of their previous lives—their "normal" lives—and thrust into a shadowy half-life where some things may be the same (now that we have toilet paper again), but many things feel as if they will never return to life as we knew it before.

Jungian psychologists refer to places like this, including the netherworld to which Persephone was abducted, as "liminal." This word comes from the Greek word *limen*, which means *threshold*. When we are in a liminal space, we are between worlds, between times, between what was and what will be, between the known and the unknown. This is never a comfortable place to be, especially not when we first arrive there. It makes us wonder if we will ever be ourselves again...our familiar selves as we had come to know and accept them. And the trickiest part is that this liminal place is usually *not* hellish. It is just...between. Time is suspended, life is suspended, reality is suspended. Yes, we do some normal things in liminal space, but it's unclear whether those things are *real*...that is, real in the same way that things felt real when we did them before.

The ancient Greeks referred to Hades, the liminal world to which Persephone was abducted, as a realm of darkest shadows...but also vast riches. When we first arrive in any liminal place of *between*, it usually feels like it is made more of shadows than riches. But the Greeks would have said, and one specific Greek did famously say, that we feel that way because we are awakening to the truth that we have been living among shadows all along... and only mistaking them for reality. This leads us to a fifth myth, again from ancient Greece, and not exactly a myth this time, but close enough to count as one. I'm talking about a timeless story that the philosopher Plato recounted in his best-known book, *The Republic*.[154] Technically, it is called "The Allegory of the Cave," and it may be the most crucial story of any that Plato created.

It seems important to begin by saying that Plato did not start out as a philosopher. He was the son of a prominent Greek family that wanted

154.Plato. *The Republic*. Translated by Desmond Lee. New York: Penguin Classics, 2007, pp 240-248.

him to become a statesman. But when his beloved teacher Socrates was condemned to a political death by forced suicide, Plato pivoted his life and became a leading educator in Greek philosophy. Using stories and dialogues, as Socrates had, Plato articulated his views of the human mind and social consciousness in a way that has transcended time and social revolutions. Plato's "Academy" was the first university in the Western world, and it endured for three hundred years. What's more, Plato's body of work is the only ancient canon to survive intact through the 2,400 years since it was written.

Now, let's take a look at the liminal netherworld of Plato's Cave...

In this subterranean realm, all people are seated and bound, with their necks and backs resting against a low wall so that they are looking at the back wall of the Cave. Far behind them, at the opening of the Cave, there is an enormous fire that burns continually. And between the low wall against which they rest their backs and the burning fire, there are scores of people who move back and forth, carrying an infinite variety of objects. The seated people cannot see the objects nor the people carrying them, but they can see the shadows that the objects cast against the back wall of the Cave. For the seated people, these dancing shadows comprise the whole of reality.

Plato asks us to consider a single person among the seated people—a person who somehow gets free of the bonds and is able to stand up and look directly back at the opening of the Cave. The person now sees the fire and the people who carry the objects. The person suddenly realizes that what had previously seemed to be "reality" were only the shadows of actual objects—*real* shadows, but shadows nonetheless. And it also becomes clear that those objects are being carried by *real* people who are not bound to the wall, as this person was.

At first, the light of the fire is so bright that it hurts the eyes of the newly-freed person. In fact, the person is tempted to sit back down and resume looking at the shadows on the back wall, because the excruciating light of the fire and mind-blowing fact of a three-dimensional world are almost too overwhelming to bear. But in the story, the person decides to persist and continue exploring. Venturing closer to the fire burning at the cave's entryway, it becomes clear that there is an even brighter light on the outside of the door of the Cave. Eventually, the person gathers enough courage to step through this door and into the outer world.

If the three-dimensional objects and the fire of the Cave were overwhelming, we can imagine how shocking the world of landscapes and objects and animals and people must be to the formerly-bound person. And the sun! So much light that it cannot be borne! At first, the person can only stand in the shade, mostly with closed eyes. But gradually, it becomes possible to explore that outer world with eyes open, and even to gaze very briefly at the sun. Once this becomes the person's new reality, there is no returning to the old consciousness of the Cave.

The question, in fact, is whether the person will return to the Cave at all. It is so tempting to remain in this brilliant, colorful, solid world! And the bound people of the Cave now seem so ignorant and brutish, in comparison to the place where the person has arrived in body and mind. But in the end, the person decides that there is a moral obligation to share this new awareness with those who are still bound in the Cave. And for that reason, the person returns.

It would be nice to think that those who are still bound in the Cave would welcome the news that this enlightened person brings back from the outer world. But in fact, many of the bound people reject the story that the person brings to them about light and color and solid forms. The shadows on the wall are familiar to the bound people, and some of them do not want to live with a different reality, particularly a reality whose exploration requires an experience of pain. And so the person is faced with a lifelong dilemma between educating those who wish to engage the outer world, and simultaneously accepting those who reject the outer world and cling to the shadows dancing on the back of the Cave as the sum of their reality.

Some of us have experienced this pandemic time as an encounter with Plato's Cave. Or perhaps it feels as if our lives before the pandemic had elements of Plato's Cave woven throughout them. We previously considered our lives to be as real as rocks, when in fact we were witnessing a shadow dance that imitated life but did not actualize it. We were living an "as if" life. Death can make the distinction between "as if" and "really is" blazingly clear for us, in a way that few other things can. The poet Mary Oliver famously asked us to observe that death comes to us inevitably, and always before we would wish it. And that fact, she said, is what invites each of us to consider what it is we want to make of our unique existences.[155]

155. Oliver, Mary. "The Summer Day" in *New and Selected Poems*. New York: Beacon Press, 1993.

Today, as the vaccines give us hope for expansion, many of us in the more privileged countries of the world are wrestling with what it means to "re-open," to emerge from the shadow worlds of our caves. Some people are erupting from their caves without appearing to have given much consideration to what has the most "reality"—that is, what has deepest meaning in their lives. For those people, the shadow dances will just resume in their old way, if they ever stopped at all. (It is hard to resist comparing Plato's dancing shadows to the images of pseudo-life that mesmerize us on our electronic screens.)

However, if the things that are being expressed today in public venues have any validity, there are many people who are now seeking the kind of meaning that can guide them toward whatever makes life worth living to them. Some people want to spend more time with others, some want to spend less. Some people have discovered interests, even passions, that they had never realized could give so much meaning to their lives, even as they also realize that the things they pursued in the past now seem unworthy of all that effort. Each person has had the opportunity during this time of descent to look around, to see the actual objects that cast the shadows on the wall, and to perceive the fire that makes all shadows possible. This is a time in which awakenings can happen, new decisions can be made, new possibilities can be considered, and new paths may be explored.

This discovery of a new reality that was previously unseen takes us to the real meaning of the word *apocalypse*. We commonly think of this word as an end-of-the-world scenario—dreadful beasts, fabulous monsters, and deadly Horsemen...including Pestilence. But the actual meaning of *apocalypse* (ἀποκάλυψις) is "the revealing of that which has been previously hidden." Yes, the new things that are revealed may implicate the ending of some things from the time before. But this is *not* the end of the entire world. Rather, it is the beginning of a new age in the world. These newly-revealed things come from the seeds of truth that certain people throughout history have discovered during their descents in a pandemic time, seeds that they have planted and nurtured into their post-pandemic lives. It is not everyone's choice (or ability) to do this, just as it was not everyone's choice (or ability) to leave Plato's Cave. But for those who make this choice during the coronavirus pandemic, it will certainly lead to consequences of profound meaning.

#6—Consciously or not, we and our world will be changed by this pandemic. The only question is whether or not we will participate in that change and embrace its effects.

We delight in the beauty of the butterfly,
but rarely admit the changes it has gone through
to achieve that beauty.
– Maya Angelou[156]

When she transformed into a butterfly,
the caterpillars spoke not of her beauty,
but of her weirdness.
They wanted her to change back
into what she always had been.
But she had wings.
– Dean Jackson[157]

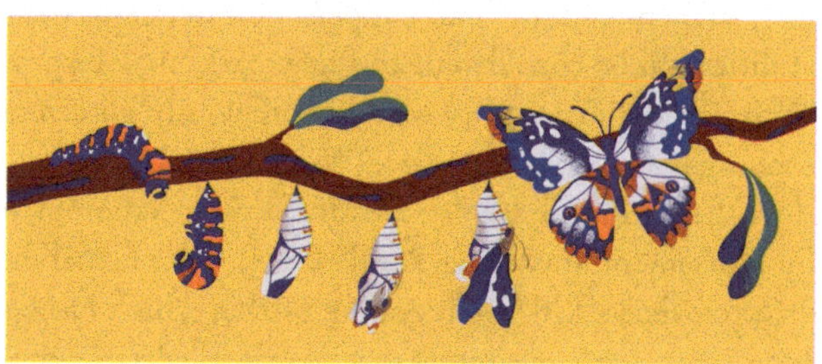

(Shutterstock)

The ancient Greeks considered the butterfly to be the most appropriate symbol for the human soul, just as they considered Persephone to be the divine patroness of the soul. They held these beliefs because all these entities—Persephone, the butterfly, and the soul—demonstrate a stunning

156. There is no identifiable source for this oft-cited quote. The best theory is that Angelou produced it when she worked as a greeting card writer for Hallmark. (Yes, really.)

157. Jackson, Dean. *The Poetry of Oneness*. Createspace Independent Publishing Platform, 2013. ISBN 1493564803

capacity for transformation. As we contemplate the ways in which the coronavirus pandemic might be changing us and our world, it seems wise to follow the Greeks' ancient wisdom and study these models of profound transformation in myth and nature.

We are not told how Persephone accomplished her astonishing transformation from being a victim of sexual abduction to reigning as the Queen of Hades. And modern psychology is still bumping around among its hypotheses about how a human soul achieves profound transformation in the course of a lifetime. But we know quite a bit about the transformation from caterpillar to butterfly, so let's allow Nature be our guide on this portion of the journey, as she has so often been throughout this book.

When a caterpillar spins a cocoon or molts into a chrysalis, it is creating a container that is simultaneously a tomb and a womb. The creature in caterpillar form will cease to exist during the course of its metamorphosis; it will literally digest its own body to create the nourishing "soup" that will enable the butterfly to be born. But the caterpillar does not digest *all* of itself into the soup. It leaves intact a host of tiny cell bundles from which the butterfly will be formed. Each of these little cell bundles, which have been given the poetic name "imaginal discs," carries the blueprint for a portion of the butterfly's body. During the time spent in its cocoon or chrysalis, the butterfly creates itself, using the digested soup and the imaginal discs that were left behind by the self-sacrificing caterpillar. And in the end, the butterfly emerges as a creature that appears to be entirely new...but is actually composed entirely of its caterpillar.

When we are abducted by a pandemic into a dark netherworld like those of Persephone or Dante, it usually brings us restriction, isolation, dread, uncertainty, grief, and/or despair. However, we might consider that we, too, are entering a chrysalis—a tomb and a womb in which we can retain the essential stuff of our beings, but in which we can also be transformed into a version of ourselves that is essentially new and remarkably different, a version of ourselves that will allow us to live in ways that we could not have lived before.

Plato does not tell us how it originally happens that one Cave person stands up and turns away from the dancing shadows. He does not say why it is that this one person is able to tolerate the pain and fear that are ignited by the real world. He does not explain why this particular person decides to go back and share the news with the people who remain bound in the cave, even when they seem so primitive, and even when they reject the gift of truth. These are mysteries that Plato has left for those of us in the millennia that have succeeded him, just as Persephone's transformation in Hades has remained a mystery throughout those same millennia. But we can imagine that there is something in the story of the caterpillar's metamorphosis into butterfly that applies to these stories—a liquifying of one's former self, a preservation of one's essential "imaginal discs," and a reconstitution into a new version of oneself. But this time...with wings.

It is too early to say what any of us might look and act like as post-pandemic butterflies. Maybe those changes will never be describable in words. Maybe they will only be felt in the transformed individual's heart and soul, and only expressed with new gestures and shapes of living. Of course, many people will not have undergone any metamorphosis at all. Not every caterpillar survives the cocoon or chrysalis. Not every caterpillar is even able to create a container of transformation. That is no one's fault. There is no judgment in the kaleidoscope of Nature. There are too many factors operating in each individual story to permit us the audacity of judging its outcome. We have only the individual stories to witness, ours from the inside and others' from the outside. Most importantly, each of us has our own story to consider in terms of what we were before and what we are now. Caterpillar to butterfly—each of us constant in our substance and yet profoundly different in our manifested being.

The same is true of the meaningful changes that this pandemic might precipitate in the world's societies. The societal metamorphoses will probably be too slow, subtle, and complex to allow our individual minds and mortal bodies to grasp them from the perspective of this time and place. To paraphrase Emerson Pugh again, "If the world were so simple that we could understand it, we would be so simple that we couldn't." But we have already seen that this pandemic has awakened many of us to the facts that:

1. The density of our populations is likely to trigger more pandemics, and to make the pandemics we trigger more severe and deadly.
2. For this reason, there can no longer be such a thing as a "localized" pandemic, especially if the pathogen is airborne. We are too numerous and too mobile to restrict airborne pathogens to a contained locale.
3. Our responses to global problems, especially those that are fundamentally occurring in nature, must be immediate, collaborative, and equitable. Nothing reminds us that we are a global village like an environmental catastrophe, especially a lethal pandemic.

4. The primacy of Nature is announcing itself collectively, as well as personally. The Earth's declarations of our environmental imbalances are accelerating, people's assertions of their biological identities are proliferating, and Nature's demonstrations of global vulnerability, such as this pandemic, are increasing in frequency and intensity.
5. The reality of these changes is verified by the ferocious human resistance to them. Important social change never happens without a regressive backlash, and the more important the change, the more intense and regressive the backlash. It would be lovely if this pandemic were to ignite universal and unopposed progress on the natural issues of environmental health, population balance, biological equity for individuals and groups, and harmonic relations with the microscopic world. Not in this lifetime, my friends. Resistance may be futile, but it is also inevitable during times of major transition.[158]

Of course, as I wander through this list of possible social consequences from the coronavirus pandemic, I must remember that the major social consequences from the historical pandemics were so profound and evolutionary that it would have been impossible for anyone to have clearly foreseen them while the pandemic was still active. For example...

Could Justinian's subjects have imagined the mentality of independent nations that became deeply rooted in the European psyche five hundred years after their plague?

Could the devoted followers of the medieval Catholic church have imagined a world, little more than a century after the onslaught of the Black Death, in which humanism and science could flourish and the Church would no longer hold primacy in people's lives?

Could the pre-Columbian nations of Mesoamerica have predicted a world in which their perpetual wars and blood-soaked rituals would be ended for the sake of solidarity against the multiple dangers—political and biological—that threatened their survival as a people?

Could the combatants of 1918 have imagined a world in which the death count from their influenza pandemic would be eventually tallied in the tens of millions, and the search for its instigator would lead to a revolution in vaccination and epidemic control?

158. For example: Leahy, Peter J. and Allan Mazur. "The rise and fall of public opposition in specific social movements." *Social Studies of Science*, Vol. 10, No. 3 (1980) 259-284. https://doi.org/10.1177/030631278001000301

The answer to all these questions is, of course, "No, they could not. Those notions were utterly beyond what was conceivable for each of those peoples." Therefore, we must assume that the most important and meaningful social consequences from the coronavirus pandemic are equally inconceivable for us. And how comforting that is! How inspiring! Yes, it's too bad that most of us will never live to see those consequences, but it's exciting to imagine what that inconceivably new world—that global butterfly—will be like.

Historically, pandemics have forced humans
to break with the past and imagine their world anew.
This one is no different.
It is a portal, a gateway between one world and the next.
We can choose to walk through it,
dragging the carcasses of our prejudice and hatred,
our avarice, our data banks and dead ideas,
our dead rivers and smoky skies behind us.
Or we can walk through lightly, with little luggage,
ready to imagine another world.
And ready to fight for it.
– Arundhati Roy [159]

Concluding...and Continuing

What a piece of work is a man!
How noble in reason, how infinite in faculties,
in form and moving how express and admirable,
in action how like an angel, in apprehension how like a god!
The beauty of the world, the paragon of animals!
And yet, to me, what is this quintessence of dust?
– William Shakespeare, *Hamlet*, II.ii

159. Roy, Arundhati. "The Pandemic is a Portal" *The Financial Times*, April 3, 2020. https://www.ft.com/content/10d8f5e8-74eb-11ea-95fe-fcd274e920ca

We are stardust,
Billion-year-old carbon.
We are golden,
Caught in the devil's bargain.
And we've got to get ourselves
back to the garden.
– Joni Mitchell [160]

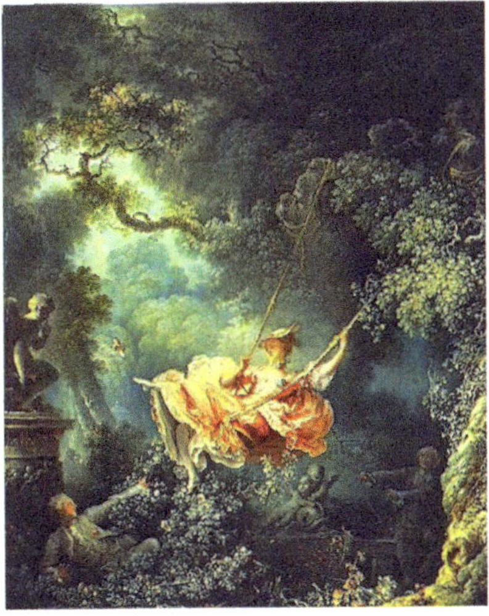

The Swing, Jean-Honoré Fragonard (1867) (Wikimedia)

There is no adequate way to close this narrative, and that is only natural because the curtain has not yet come down on this pandemic drama. Indeed, there is no way that a line of words, of any length or majesty, can do justice to what we have suffered and lost in any of our wars with pandemic disease. Much has been achieved, and much has even been won, but at an unspeakable cost.

Death can be our greatest teacher, humbling us and reminding us that for all our astonishing accomplishments as simple bipeds on this grand planet, at the end of it all, "nothing can we call our own but death." And yet, and yet... Before we surrender to our inevitable citizenship in that far

160.Mitchell, Joni. Woodstock. Words and Music by Joni Mitchell. Copyright © 1969 Crazy Crow Music. Copyright renewed. All Rights Administered Worldwide by Reservoir Media Management, Inc. All Rights Reserved. Used by Permission. Reprinted by Permission of Hal Leonard LLC.

country beyond life, there is this glorious moment of breath in which we can shine like golden stardust, burning with the audacity to do *some*thing before our moment ends. Striving to do something that, if nothing else, has meaning for the person doing it.

The psychiatrist Elizabeth Kübler-Ross has proclaimed that we humans greet death with a combination of denial, anger, bargaining, depression, and acceptance. Although she originally talked about those feelings as linear "stages," most therapists now consider them ingredients in a complex emotional mixture. But Kübler-Ross left out what Carl Jung would have declared to be the most important ingredient of all in our encounters with death. Jung believed that death will bring us no more than brute suffering unless we can derive from it a sense of *meaning*.

The discovery of meaning is a very personal thing. We do not find meaning in a book, no matter how earnestly the author tries to illuminate her subject. We only find meaning in the privacy of our own hearts, after we have learned some facts and gained some perspective and thought our own thoughts and felt our own feelings. After all that, our unique sense of meaning will come to us, usually in its own sweet time and often taking us by complete surprise. Because meaning itself is a very mysterious thing. We know it for what it is, but only when we have it in hand. A personal sense of meaning allows us to place our experience in a context that both contains it and liberates it, with perspective and illumination. Meaning may not provide a solution, but it does provide us with a handle that we can use to hold onto all of the incomprehensible things that will otherwise confuse, elude, and frighten us. And once we find that anchoring grip on our experience, no one can take it away from us.

Among all the facts and perspectives that you have encountered in this book, I hope you will have encountered some few things that will ignite your thoughts and feelings, some few things that will give you a sense of personal meaning for the life-and-death drama of the coronavirus pandemic. Each flicker of meaning that a reader derives will be like the beating wings of a butterfly—apparently fragile and fleeting but, according to Chaos Theory, capable of changing the weather on a global scale. For the pestilence-slain multitudes of the past, for the pestilence-vulnerable multitudes of the future, and for every pestilence-afflicted soul today, our discoveries of meaning will serve as beacons of light in the recurring darkness of pandemic disease.

♦ ♦ ♦

The best final words for any large story are those of a playwright or a poet. I have relied greatly on the words of William Shakespeare in this book, but I believe that Shakespeare would approve of the following words to end this journey. They were written by T. S. Eliot during a literal firestorm of war that was rather like a pandemic—a cataclysm of death in which Eliot seemed to use his own search for meaning as a beacon through a fearsome night and into a redemptive dawn.

Every phrase and every sentence is an end and a beginning,
Every poem an epitaph. And any action
Is a step to the block, to the fire, down the sea's throat
Or to an illegible stone: and that is where we start.

We die with the dying:
See, they depart, and we go with them.
We are born with the dead:
See, they return, and bring us with them.
The moment of the rose and the moment of the yew-tree
Are of equal duration...

We shall not cease from exploration
And the end of all our exploring
Will be to arrive where we started
And know the place for the first time...

Quick now, here, now, always—
A condition of complete simplicity
(Costing not less than everything)
And all shall be well and
All manner of thing shall be well
When the tongues of flames are in-folded
Into the crowned knot of fire
And the fire and the rose are one.

– T. S. Eliot[161]

161. Eliot, T. S. From "Little Gidding" in *Four Quartets* by T. S. Eliot. Copyright © 1936 by Houghton Mifflin Harcourt Publishing Company, renewed 1964 by T. S. Eliot. Copyright © 1940, 1941, 1942 by T. S. Eliot, renewed 1968, 1969, 1970 by Esme Valerie Eliot. Used by permission of HarperCollins Publishers and Faber & Faber Ltd.

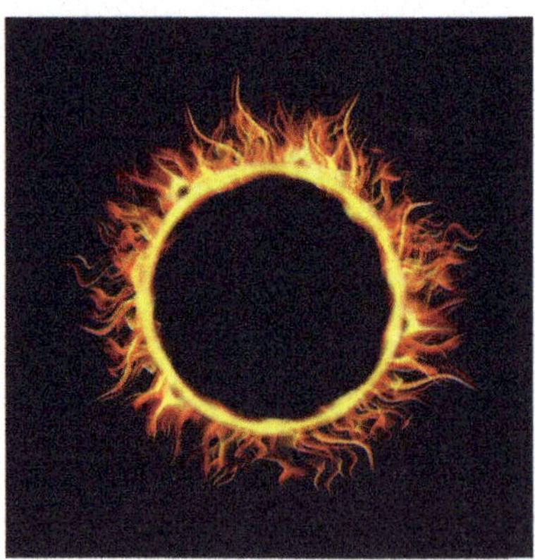

Depiction of the corona ("crown") during an eclipse of our sun (Shutterstock)

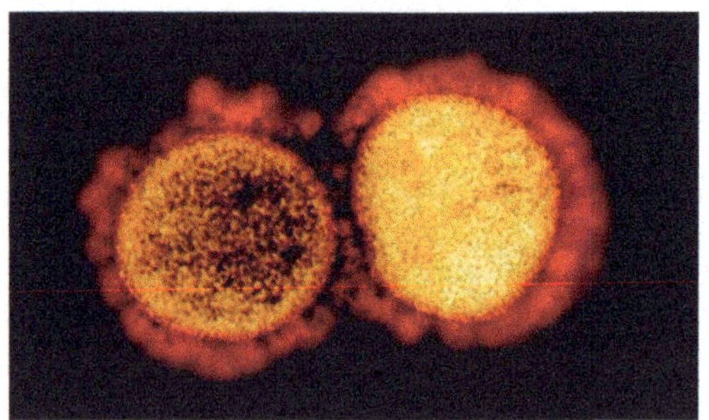

Electron microscope photo of the novel coronavirus (NIAID)

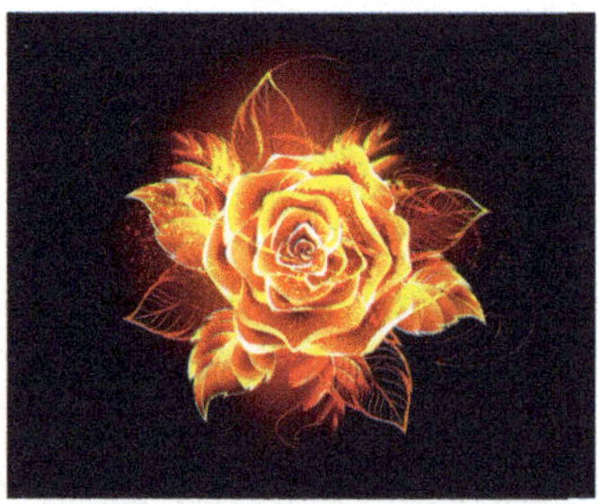

Depiction of the "crowned knot of fire" when "the fire and the rose are one" (Shutterstock)

Acknowledgements

They say that writing is a solitary endeavor, but that's like saying that a tree is a solitary being. Without soil and sun and water and air, a tree will never be more than a dead twig. So it is with a writer and the book she creates.

The following people have been my soil and sun, my water and air. Without their inspiring, nourishing, and sustaining contributions, I could never have survived the telling of this pestilential tale. In myriad ways, they replenished my quavering spirit, my vulnerable body, my inconstant resolve, and my tattered sense of humor. There aren't enough words of gratitude to repay the generosity of these elemental supporters. I only hope that they will find sufficient worth in this fully grown beast to justify all they have devoted to its birthing.

To **Chris Coleman**, who was the first to insist, beyond all reason, that such a book should be written and that I should be the one to write it. You read the very first versions of the very first chapters, Chris, and you continued to encourage me even after you completed that daunting task. I offer you my deepest gratitude for the shining mirror of your regard. It is you who helped me to realize that the best way to make meaning of anything, especially something as vast, terrifying, and incomprehensible as a global pandemic, is by telling its dramatic story, just as courageous theater artists have been doing for millennia.

To **Susan Paidhrin, M.A., Ph.D.**, my beloved mentor and cherished friend, who immediately and enthusiastically offered to serve as a primary reader for the manuscript, and who eventually became my main advisor for its content and editing. I will remain in your debt, heart and soul, for all of my days. Your starlit counsel has always been as wise as it is loving, and your breadth of knowledge will forever astound me. But this task was surely among your most formidable works of guidance, education, and encouragement. The final copy editor referred to this beast as "a polished piece of work," and that high praise belongs to you, Susan.

To **Nina Mahaffey, M.A., L.M.F.T., R.N.**, my dear friend and one of the most perceptive intellectuals I've ever met. You cheerfully agreed to serve as my second primary reader when the manuscript's first draft was complete, and your analysis gave me crucial considerations for future revisions. I am certain that this beast will never meet a more incisive evaluator of its major premises than you, Nina, and that has given me a confidence that I never could have achieved on my own. My thanks as well to you and your brilliant husband **Patrick Mahaffey, Ph.D.**, for inviting me to speak on this topic to the students at Pacifica Graduate Institute, which gave me the opportunity to fly my dark kite in the bright wind of their regard.

To **Jean Shinoda Bolen, M.D.**, who received my newly birthed manuscript and carried it into the world with a fierce determination that has filled me with grateful wonder. No newborn being could ever have a more powerful and devoted godmother than you, Jean. The fact that this particular newborn carries a story of global suffering and fundamental meaning makes her future especially worthy of your potent advocacy. My beast is extremely fortunate to have you as her champion...and so am I. Indeed, Jean, my gratitude is so far beyond words that it can only be spoken fully with my heart.

To **Julie Harrelson**, who heard more about the novel coronavirus, the coronavirus pandemic, and pandemic history in general — fact by dreadful fact, discovery by bewildering discovery, story by horrific story — than anyone else who had the mischance to wander near me during the past two and a half years. No matter how dismal the news of the day might have been, no matter how we trembled at the latest statistics of illness and death, no matter how ominous the future seemed, you were always ready to hear me out, asking me illuminating questions and making me laugh, even at death. Everyone needs a stalwart companion for a descent into the Inferno, and no one could have served in that role better than you, Julie. Not even Dante's Beatrice.

To **Elisabeth Baerg Hall, M.D.**, my brilliant and generous friend of the medical persuasion, who spent countless hours helping me understand the dizzying complexities of infection, contagion, and the human immune system...and to understand it well enough so that I could describe it in accessible terms for the non-scientifically inclined. My clarity is the result of *your* clarity, Elisabeth. And let me remind you that *you* were the first person to say, long before the researchers did, that Covid-19 was a *vascular* disease...and you were *right*! Thank you as well for introducing my Chapters 2 and 3 to your dear friend and expert colleague **Jack Kliman, M.D.** The two of you reviewed my science carefully, so that I could sound far more knowledgeable about virology, immunology, and infectious diseases than

I really am. My profound thanks to you both for being the scientific and ethical wind beneath my wings. (And to be sure, any remaining errors are entirely my own!)

To **Dave O'Neal**, the editor of my first book, who was my insightful and forthright mentor in the creation of that entity. It has been nearly thirty years since we embarked on that journey, Dave, but during the writing and publishing of *this* beast, I have leaned upon the inner voice of your wisdom and reassurance more times than I can count, and the memories of our discussions have guided me to safe harbor, even now. I cherished your counsel when I first received it, but it's possible that I cherish it even more today, when I have had no actual Dave O at my shoulder...only the memory of your wise (and witty) words in my heart. I hope you will perceive the best of what you taught me in what you find on these pages.

To **Kate Carroll deGutes** and **Yussef El-Guindi**, my two dear friends of literary elegance and accomplishment who have educated and encouraged me as a Writer, which I had never before considered myself to be. You have stood as shining examples of what I admire most in Writers — courage, eloquence, tenacity, and strong values. And when appropriate, you have offered me the bounty of your advice, gathered from your hard-won years of successful experience. I only hope that what you are and how you write has ignited a bit of the same things in my writing...and in me.

To **Susannah Mars, Marissa Wolf, Frances Barnes, Kate Carroll deGutes, Sue Fahrbach**, and **Nola Horton-Jones**, the intrepid friends who agreed to apply their keen minds and professional perspectives (theatrical, literary, and pragmatic, respectively) to the bold notions that I have put forth in this book. A writer always prefers to have discerning friends point out her errors of fact and logic, rather than making a fool of herself in public print. Having passed muster with all of you — whip-smart and uncompromising as you are — I feel I can now safely face the public without being found guilty of unpardonable foolishness.

To **Rick Lewis** and **Gavin Hoffman**, my beloved friends and my masters in the theater arts, I offer my infinite gratitude for your having sustained my soul with the gifts of Sondheim and Shakespeare, respectively. It would have been impossible to pursue my search for meaning in the midst of contagion, if I had not been able to experience with you, week by viral week, the supreme joy of playing with some of the best toys in the theatrical sandbox.

Your lessons reminded me about how and why some people have been able to pursue their campaign against Pestilence; sometimes we fight for life in the depths of despair because of art and meaning and love, and the joy of bringing them together in our bodies. Thank you, Rick and Gavin, for sharing that knowledge with me so that I could feel it for myself, especially on the darkest days.

To **Mike Louaillier, Pamela Lumpkins, Cathy Rote, David Meyers,** and **Marilyn Reynolds,** my champions in the realms of finance and the law. Everything I have accomplished stands upon the solid foundations of your excellent judgments and sincere devotions to my well-being. In addition to being gifted stewards in your areas of expertise, you have also been cherished friends, supporting my diverse endeavors even when they were distant from your own familiar grounds. And that is, to me, the hallmark of real champions. Thank you for being mine.

To **Pam Kulcinski**, my partner in the management of every aggravating detail in my life. We have often joked that the secret of our success is our ability to position our Swiss cheese brains so that only the tiny mistakes fall through. But really, Pam, it is your diligence and devotion, enhanced by mutual respect and affection, that have kept me upright and on schedule.

To **Richa Uppal, M.D., Elizabeth Morgan, M.D., John Kojis, D.C., Marina Zaré, D.C., Cheryl Veach**, and **Kelly Nguen**, my gifted physical caregivers. Writing a book like this entails one kind of risk to a writer's psyche, but more importantly, it entails literal risk to the writer's soft animal body, which must digest and metabolize the energies that glue together every horrific image and despairing statistic. The six of you have kindly and courageously cared for my loyal body while she and I have walked the gruesome road of humanity's deadliest catastrophes. I owe to you all my surprising good health, my blessed sense of well-being, and, probably, my life.

To the **Kuiper family — Mikaela, Ron,** and **Paula** — who have miraculously assumed the burden of owning, stewarding, and nurturing the FarmHill Equestrian Center. You three remarkable souls, along with the cherished community of support that includes **Alexis Young, Cheryl McGuire, Dr. Anne Marie Ray, Dr. Meg Brinton,** and **Scott Uskoski**, have made it possible for me to complete this project. Without your deep dedication to my beloved beasts, I could never have mustered the inner strength that was required to bring *this* beast to life.

To **Dolly Dee Dunbar** and **Ravyn Dunbar**, who have devoted their excellent and sincere care to my dear home and feline family. Without your presence in our lives, I would have no safe haven from which to launch my words into the world. All animals love the two of you, and with good reason, and that includes the soft animal of my own body/soul. Thank you for the comforting laps, literal and metaphorical, that you provide in my life!

To the masterful team coordinated by **Bradley Communications Corporation**, including **Cristina Smith** of Steve Harrison AuthorSuccess, **Valerie Costa** of Costa Creative Services, **Christy Day** and **Maggie McLaughlin** of Constellation Book Services, **Steve Scholl** of the WaterStone Agency, and **Kimberlie Cruse** of Steve Harrison Unforgettable Speaker Training, I extend my profound gratitude. You have brought to this endeavor the formidable resources of the publishing world at its best — that is, expertise devoted to my personal values and my specific goals for this book. I thank you all for your sincere dedication to my work. A writer and her book can only experience success with a team like you to make it happen.

To the gracious technical wizards at **DogPaw Studio**, led by **Chijo Takeda** — who together conjured a beautiful website out of thin air, client ignorance, and technical brilliance — I offer my endless admiration and deepest thanks. You have managed to create, with elegance, efficiency, and gentle humor, a website that conveys much of my essence and a mountain of information. It takes a certain kind of magic to transform a client's dread into pure delight, and you have made that magic for me.

And I want to thank the friends who have loyally sustained me, sometimes without knowing or saying anything explicit about this beast, but simply by giving me your palpable support and enduring love because you knew that I was doing Something Very Hard. You always let me know that you were there to see me through this dark journey, all the way to the welcome dawn. You include **Sue Fahrbach, J. Roxane Russell, Susannah Mars, Jean Bolen, Nola Horton-Jones, Troy Brown, Camille King, Rick Lewis, Gavin Hoffman,** and of course, **Chris Coleman.** My heart to all of yours in grateful friendship.

Finally, it is with immense gratitude that I want to acknowledge **Orvis "Orv" Harrelson, M.D.**, who dedicated his long and distinguished career to the practice of public health medicine. Because Dr. Harrelson was a lifetime learner, and because my topic piqued his curiosity, he asked to read my manuscript in October 2021, less than three months before his death at the age of 94. It was primarily in response to Dr. Harrelson's urgent directive that *Hollow Crown of Fire* be made public that I acquiesced to the notion of bringing this daunting beast into the light of published day. If Orv thought my beast was worth a public viewing, then who was I to argue with his lifelong experience? Rest in wisdom, Orv, and may this book fulfill your vision for its destiny.

Index

About the Author

BARBARA E. HORT, Ph.D. has maintained a private practice in Portland, Oregon for over 30 years, working primarily with the psychological approach developed by the psychoanalyst Carl Jung. Her practice has been deepened by her postgraduate work with the Jungian analysts Jean Shinoda Bolen M.D. and Marion Woodman, both of whom have emphasized the role of the Feminine and Nature in their approach to Jungian practice. For the past decade, Dr. Hort has collaborated with theater director Chris Coleman to develop the theatrical practice of *psychodramaturgy*, in which she provides material on the psychological dynamics of a play that can be used by its producing artists to enhance their theatrical storytelling (www.psychodramaturgy.com). Previously, Dr. Hort served on the faculties of Reed College in Portland, Oregon and Washington State University - Vancouver, publishing numerous academic research articles in the fields of social and developmental psychology. In addition to *Hollow Crown of Fire*, Dr. Hort is the author of *Unholy Hungers: Encountering the Psychic Vampire in Ourselves and Others* (Boston: Shambhala, 1996). Dr. Hort can be contacted at www.BarbaraHort.com

Made in the USA
Columbia, SC
11 February 2023